DEDICATION

To you, the woman who has chosen to read our book and embark on a new journey toward aligning with the best version of yourself and your life.

May you uncover your vibrant and unique essence, reclaim your power, and find the courage to live with liberation, confidence, and happiness. Embrace your life with enthusiasm, free from the need for a drink.

ADVANCE PRAISE FOR *TIPSY*

Tipsy: A Woman's Self-Guided Method for Managing Alcohol is not only a book about recovery, it's a beautiful guide to self-discovery! As a clinical health psychologist, it is refreshing to find a resource that directly explains the unique female experience of substance use issues. In *Tipsy*, the authors effectively address "the seductive pull of your comfort zone," "the feminine drinking culture," and the "willingness to be vulnerable" as women bond over alcohol. No other book so aptly explores the nuances of feminine alcohol use! Inspiring, empowering, yet down to earth—this book is an ESSENTIAL TOOL for both women and any clinician who works in alcohol treatment.

Dr. Katherine T. Kelly, PhD, MSPH
Clinical Health Psychologist and Soul-Healing Specialist
Best-Selling Author of *Anxiety: Treating Body, Mind and Soul* and *Depression: Treating Body, Mind and Soul*

Clinical psychologist Alicia Lamberghini-West is the author of *Your Life, Your Way*, an ideal guide that every woman should read. And now, in her new book, *Tipsy: A Woman's Self-Guided Method for Managing Alcohol*, co-authored with Pilar Karlen Triplett, she goes even further, advising women who are not necessarily alcoholics but would like to control their drinking, how to lead more liberated lives. Indeed, the methods she and Triplett use, and their good, solid advice to their many readers may well make them America's best and most trusted writers for women, wherever they may be on their life's journey.

Rosemary Daniell,
Author of *Secrets of the Zona Rosa: How Writing (and Sisterhood) Can Change Women's Lives,* and nine other books of poetry and prose

In my professional practice, I've noticed a concerning trend: an increasing number of women are turning to alcohol more frequently. According to the insights shared in *Tipsy*, this rise in consumption may be closely related to the numerous pressures and challenges women face in their daily lives. The book provides a comprehensive self-guided method designed to assist women in controlling their drinking habits. This approach could be highly beneficial in preventing both emotional and physical dependence on alcohol, and in helping women avoid the various negative consequences associated with excessive drinking. By addressing the root causes and offering practical strategies, this book has the potential to make a significant positive impact on many women's lives.

Edgar Galiñanes, MD
Cox Health Services Inpatient Psychiatry
Board Certified in Psychiatry and Neurology
Medical Preceptor in Psychiatry, Columbia University Medical School
(Columbia, MO)

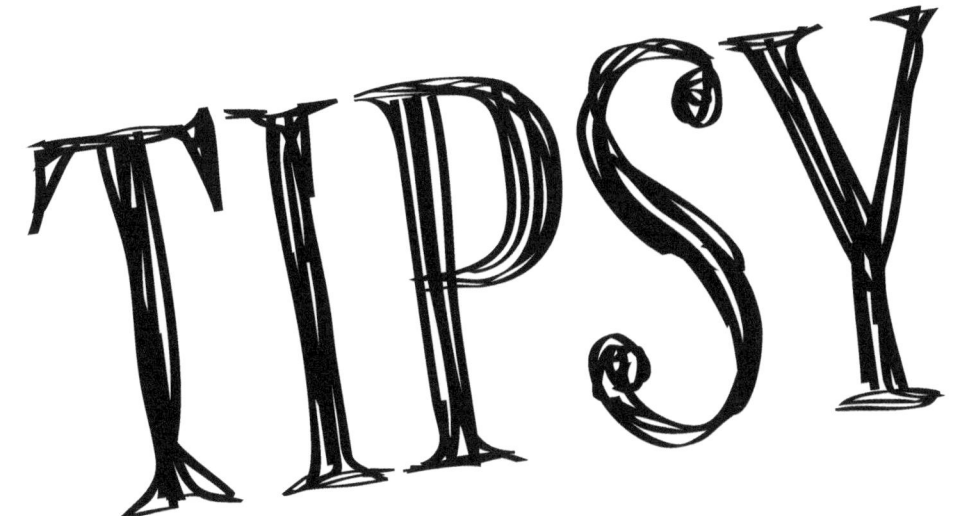

A Woman's Self-Guided Method for Managing Alcohol

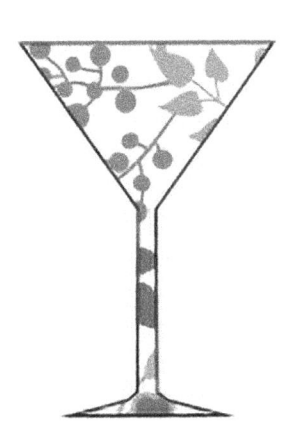

Dr. Alicia Lamberghini-West, PsyD (Author)
Pilar Karlen Triplett, Life & Health Coach (Author)
and Dr. William Triplett, MD (Contributor)

Copyright © 2025 Alicia Lamberghini-West, Pilar Karlen Triplett, William Triplett

ALL RIGHTS RESERVED

No part of this book may be translated, used, or reproduced in any form or by any means, in whole or in part, electronic or mechanical, including photocopying, recording, taping, or by any information storage or retrieval system without express written permission from the author or the publisher, except for the use in brief quotations within critical articles and reviews.

You can contact the authors through
www.tipsywoman.com

Limits of Liability and Disclaimer of Warranty:

The authors and/or publisher shall not be liable for your misuse of this material. The contents are strictly for informational and educational purposes only.

Disclaimer:

This book is intended for informational purposes only and is not a substitute for professional medical advice, diagnosis, or treatment. Always seek the advice of your physician, psychologist, or other qualified healthcare provider with any questions you may have regarding a medical or psychological condition. Never disregard professional advice or delay in seeking it because of something you have read in this book.

The information presented in this book is based on clinical observations and sources the authors believe to be reliable. However, no guarantee is made regarding the accuracy, completeness, or timeliness of the information provided. Readers are encouraged to conduct their own research and consult with appropriate professionals before making any decisions based on the information contained in this book.

The identities of individuals referenced in this book have been altered or presented in composite form to protect their privacy and confidentiality. Any resemblance to real persons, living or deceased, is purely coincidental. The content of this book is directed to educational purposes and should not be construed as representing the experiences or actions of any specific individual or group.

By making use of this book, readers acknowledge and accept these terms.

Printed and bound in the United States of America
ISBNs:
Hardback: 979-8-9917129-0-3
Paperback: 979-8-9917129-1-0
Ebook: 979-8-9917129-2-7)

CONTENTS

Preface...1
Introduction..7

Part 1: A Complicated Relationship 17
    Chapter 1: Women and Alcohol 19
    Chapter 2: Crossing the Line......................................35
    Chapter 3: What Happens When You Cross the Line.............61

Part 2: The Method—Recognizing the Problem.........95
    Chapter 4: Your Comfort Zone with Alcohol 99
    Chapter 5: The Comfort of the Victim Mentality...........105
    Chapter 6: Limiting Beliefs Keep You Stuck 109
    Chapter 7: The Negative Mindset That Prevents
        You from Changing...121

Part 3: The Method--Steps to a Solution....................125
    Chapter 8: Walk Away from That Seductive
        but Destructive Lover...127
    Chapter 9: Leave the Comfort Zone and Victim Mentality 143
    Chapter 10: Transform Limiting Beliefs into Empowering Beliefs....147
    Chapter 11: Practice a Positive Mindset........................165
    Chapter 12: Conquer the Fear Zone............................171

Chapter 13: Explore the Learning Zone 185
Chapter 14: Enter the Growth Zone...201
Chapter 15: Guidance for Specific Challenges and Situations ...209
Chapter 16: Get Past the "Just One Drink" Trap 229
Chapter 17: Build an Alcohol-Free Identity, the Key to Freedom.....241
Chapter 18: Design Your Bright Future 249
Chapter 19: The Tripod of Self-Love, Identity,
 and a Bright Future 257
Chapter 20: Looking Forward 269

Appendix..273
Quiz 1: What Is Your Relationship with Alcohol? 274
Quiz 2: Are You Part of the Feminine Drinking Culture? 278

Bibliography 281
Acknowledgements 287
About the Authors 291

PREFACE

We, Pilar and I, developed a method and consequent projects around the topic of women and alcohol. Our program is based on both of our experiences, with my background as a Doctor of Clinical Psychology, who has practiced for twenty-five years in women's issues, and a specialist in addictions and rehabilitation; and Pilar's, an Engineer and a Life and Health Coach focusing on total life transformation. We're partners in helping women to live more fulfilling, authentic lives and to think critically about what society encourages everyone to believe having a "good life" or being "a good woman" means. We also worked with a medical contributor, Dr. William Triplett, who has extensive knowledge and experience in the subject.

We, Alicia and Pilar, are mother and daughter. But more than that, we are friends and companions in life. We always say that we've walked a long road together, leaving behind our country, people, culture, and language of origin, to reach for the dreams and values that have felt true and important to us personally.

These days, something that has become synonymous with "living the good life," "enjoying life," "relaxing," and "being merry" is drinking. Alcohol has become a big part of people's daily lives and social interactions. Drinks are part of parties, holidays, vacations, and festive moments—almost as an element that's necessary and essential to celebrating at all. There are after-work drinks to relax and unwind, whether with colleagues or solo. There's having a drink with a meal or in the evenings. There are drinks on the weekends, when hanging out with family or friends, during happy hours, and on date nights. People use alcohol to amp up the fun, to be more outgoing, to enjoy life, to fit in.

Think about the times we may drink the most, such as during a breakup, divorce, empty nest period, job loss, or death of a loved one. People use alcohol to get through problems, to self-soothe and comfort, to cope with feeling bored, stressed, worried, or sad. We acknowledge the happy moments with alcohol, too. No matter what's going on with your life, alcohol makes a good partner. As long as alcohol is included, everything is fine and "normal"—and conversely, without alcohol, we're missing out! *In short, a drink is always needed—and alcohol is available everywhere.*

For many years, we, too, were convinced that all celebrations and important occasions—birthdays, weddings, holidays—had to be coupled with a good drink. We were both the typical "social drinkers." In our everyday lives, drinking was part of a "routine" that was supported by everybody. Our experiences in the two countries we've lived in, Argentina and the United States, were parallel. Drinking was part of our social culture, to the point that we believed that drinking alcohol was not only acceptable but also required; *what was not okay was deciding not to drink.*

Although we understood the sociocultural influences related to alcohol use and the subsequent health risks, we kept drinking without questioning the habit. *Why not have a drink to unwind at the end of the day? A glass of champagne when we celebrate? A glass of wine with dinner?* We had been conditioned by societal norms to think that, since we weren't alcohol-dependent, a drink or two would never harm us.

Pilar went through major life changes when she filed for divorce after twenty-one years of marriage. A year later, she became an empty nester when her son moved away to attend college. She had a big group of friends she used to go out with after work and on the weekends. One day, she had an intense epiphany and realized that she was drinking almost daily as part of her "normal" life. She was *crossing the line* with alcohol, drinking more than she wanted or intended to, and didn't like how her future would look if she continued down this path. But she didn't feel like she could discuss this with her friends, as most of them drank more than her and had no qualms about their level of consumption, feeling it was part of being "free" and "independent" as a woman.

Out of the blue, Pilar decided to become alcohol-free and told me how happy and great she felt because of this change. Shortly after, I decided to join Pilar in taking a break from alcohol. At that point, I hadn't determined if I wanted to stop drinking temporarily or permanently, and I was keeping an open mind.

We made arrangements to get together to firm up this change in our lives and compare notes. For ten days, we disconnected from our busy lives and focused on caring for our minds, bodies, and souls. We spent more time outside and moving our bodies, watching the sunrises and sunsets, cycling, and swimming. We created new routines and paid attention to our energy levels throughout the day. We read books and watched documentaries about addiction and recovery before going to bed, so our subconscious mind would stay engaged. We listened to empowering music and podcasts in the morning. We stocked our refrigerator with every kombucha flavor imaginable to replace alcoholic beverages.

Giving up alcohol was extraordinarily effortless and uncomplicated. Still, we were conscious that our temporary environment had helped us to create new routines and habits, and the challenge would be to continue after returning to our normal life. But we also had firsthand experience of how much better we felt when not drinking alcohol, and we were committed, individually and as a team, to continuing to practice this change in our daily life.

Using our professional and personal knowledge and experience, we created a plan based on the steps we took and how we responded to practical and mental challenges during our time away that we could apply to daily life. We used this work to develop AYSEN Wellness, a neutral, nonjudgmental, retreat center where we offer online and in-person help to other women interested in reconsidering their drinking.

In this book, we have replicated our program for use in an everyday environment so that anyone who wants to reconsider their drinking, either to moderate their alcohol intake or to become alcohol free, can do so. We also offer our method for reconsidering drinking via our online program.

Not long after deciding to become alcohol free, Pilar met Dr. William Triplett. They shared many interests such as practicing yoga and outdoor activities, like hiking, kayaking and stand-up paddleboarding. William was also alcohol free. Their friendship evolved into a committed relationship that led to marriage.

William became interested in our project and contributed his extensive medical expertise to this book (Chapter 3). William writes:

"For many years, I have noticed the effects that alcohol has on women's health. These effects range from subtle to dramatic, and I see them nearly every day. Despite working as a primary care physician for over twenty years, I can't remember a single time when a woman consulted me to help her with a drinking problem. *Not once.* Instead, they see me for a multitude of physical or emotional symptoms. They may be tired and aching everywhere. Many are anxious and depressed. They cannot lose weight or are otherwise unhappy with their appearance.

Frequently, they are overwhelmed with the stressors of life and unable to cope. Early in my career, I didn't pay much attention to alcohol use in my patients unless they had a disease or disorder that was a direct effect of heavy drinking. But now I recognize how even occasional binges or daily drinking more than the recommended one drink per day dramatically impacts people's health, especially in women. More alcohol intake leads to more life disruption. Now, I ask each one about their alcohol use and try to educate women about its harmful effects."

This book represents our personal views and opinions based on our lives and professional experience. We have made every attempt to provide accurate and complete information, but we acknowledge that given such a vast, nuanced topic and the uniqueness of each person's life, there may be unintentional errors or omissions, and you may find that some elements fit your situation better than others. The guidance here is informational and educational in nature, and we encourage you to apply critical thinking and verify what works for you. This book is not intended as a substitute for specific professional psychological or medical advice and should not be used to diagnose or treat any medical or psychological condition.

We use a composite narrative approach to weave together interviews and feedback from real clients (using alias names) into single stories. We've combined elements of these real-life cases so that individuals aren't identifiable in any way; however, the situations described are real.

For so many years, we interacted with alcohol as though it were relatively harmless and, what's more, a vital ingredient to socializing, celebrating, and enjoying life. But now we genuinely understand that even if alcohol can give us certain positive feelings for a while, ultimately, it will take them away and negatively impact our lives, relationships, health, finances, jobs, career opportunities, and self-esteem.

We decided to reconsider our drinking in order to engage with life more fully, free from the superficial, fake highs and typical morning lows that alcohol causes. We wrote this book for women like us, who crave more authenticity, more freedom, more self-expression, and deeper joy. *We wrote this book for you.* We want to help you to avoid the damage that results from crossing the line with alcohol and to reclaim your health.

We invite you to join us in reconsidering your drinking. It's an adventure that will have challenges but will also increase your confidence as you rise to the occasion. It will bring you greater energy and vitality, more meaningful relationships, and the opportunity to develop your full potential with joy and wholeness every day. *Are you ready? Onward!*

INTRODUCTION

Welcome! This book presents a program to guide you along a journey to reconsider your drinking.

This program has been designed especially for women, taking into account the realities, dynamics, and pressures of our lives. We respect your *free choice*—the decisions you make about your drinking and how far you choose to go on this journey are up to you. The way you manage your drinking is a reflection, in full or in part, of how you manage your life. Be confident that *the farther you go on your journey to reconsider your drinking, the more freedom, growth, and happiness you're going to gain in all areas of your life.* This is a worthy goal! We hope that this method and information we offer here supports you in making a wiser decision.

Cultural norms around women's drinking have changed dramatically over the past years. Drinking socially has become accepted in almost all situations—and even *expected* in particular circumstances. There are many societal messages and norms that reinforce this. The amount of alcohol that women drink has also increased. These changes toward further normalizing the frequency and quantity of women's drinking were consolidated and accelerated during the COVID-19 pandemic.

Maybe you're starting to realize that you might have a problem with alcohol. You question how much or how often you drink (the "flash of clarity"). Perhaps someone close to you—a significant other, family member, or friend—has commented on your alcohol intake. You may wonder what life would look like without drinking, or you have negative stereotypes about being sober (e.g., a "miserable sober"). Perhaps what used to give you *pleasure* is now starting to cause you *pain*.

What are some of the signs of a potential problem with alcohol? You may find that you need to drink an increased amount to gain the same "positive" effects and that your alcohol use has become excessive. You may break commitments with family or friends based on alcohol-related factors, such as whether alcohol will be part of an event, or due to hangovers (the set of symptoms you experience because of overdrinking). You may find that drinking affects your relationships, both personal and professional. Productivity in your job may start to decline and you may make more mistakes, with short- and long-term consequences.

The more we drink, the more we're at risk for health problems, including hypertension (leading to heart problems), liver disease, cancer, cognitive impairments, and unhealthy body weight. Plus, there are the legal issues that can result from drinking, especially when it comes to driving.

If any of this sounds familiar to you, you may think that, sooner or later, one way or another, *you'll get your alcohol intake under control*. Many people think this way, and it's a shockingly stubborn illusion, because the truth is that alcohol is extremely addictive and harmful to our health. It's easy to develop a psychological dependence on alcohol.

Crossing the Line

Current dietary guidelines suggest that adults can "choose not to drink or to drink in moderation."[1] For women, moderate intake is considered

---

1. "Drinking Levels and Patterns Defined" 2024, *National Institute on Alcohol Abuse and Alcoholism* (NIAAA).

to be one alcoholic drink[2] or less per day; heavy drinking is usually defined as consuming four or more drinks on any day or eight or more alcoholic drinks per week; while binge drinking refers to four or more drinks in about two hours. Excessive alcohol use includes patterns of alcohol consumption such as heavy drinking and binge drinking.

We use the term "crossing the line" to refer to:
- Social drinking that goes beyond moderate alcohol intake.
- Drinking more than the number of drinks you intend or want to have.
- Always finding a reason or occasion to drink.
- When alcohol is an ever-present component of your life.
- When drinking is the usual or only way you can socialize with others, cope with problems, or enjoy good moments.—This is a red flag for psychological dependence on alcohol.

Most women who are questioning their alcohol use *want to change*, but they have a hard time *imagining their life without alcohol*. We live in a culture that normalizes drinking for women, whether to cope with stress and the challenges of life ("mommy wine culture," "wine o'clock") or to socialize and fit in with others. Almost all informal gatherings and social events—including those specifically for women—are organized around drinking: girls' nights, brunches, lunches, dinners, bachelorette parties, and even baby showers.

There are many *social pressures* related to drinking. People who decide to moderate alcohol use or stop drinking altogether often feel excluded or mocked or fear that they're missing out. Sometimes people who drink *do* exclude nondrinkers because they fear being judged by them. People who reconsider their drinking also worry that others

---
2. A standard drink is the equivalent of five ounces of wine (about 12% alcohol), or twelve ounces of beer (about 5% alcohol), or 1.5 ounces distilled spirits (about 40% alcohol).

around them will misinterpret this to mean they lack self-control or were abusing alcohol. It can seem easier to continue drinking than to manage other people's questions and expectations.

If you've picked up this book, you're here with us because something inside you is calling for change. You recognize that something about your drinking right now isn't really as you want it to be, and you're looking for a different approach. In this book, we'll help you to reconsider your drinking as part of your journey of growth, freedom, and discoveries, culminating in wholeness and happiness.

A Seductive but Destructive Lover

Ann Dowsett Johnston[3] and Caroline Knapp[4] wrote about the intimate bond between women and alcohol. We continue and expand their ideas by looking at our personal relationship with drinking as a romance in which our lover, *Alcohol,* is attractive, enchanting, and seductive but astonishingly destructive. As a lover, drinking has unique characteristics:

- *Drink is charming.* You may feel that you look outgoing and have fun when you're drinking. Social, romantic, and family events and celebrations look fabulous when alcohol is present. The opposite happens as well: If you're not with your lover, you might feel bored. Dry gatherings are far from looking like fun parties.
- *Drink is possessive.* It's all or nothing. Either you're drinking and feeling your best. Or you're on a break and feel lame, excluded, and stressed out.

---
3. Ann Dowsett Johnston, *Drink: The Intimate Relationship between Women and Alcohol* (Harper Wave, 2013).
4. Caroline Knapp, *Drinking: A Love Story* (New York: The Dial Press, 1996).

- *Drink is not a good partner to you.* It lets you down when it comes to taking ownership of your life. It's always someone or something else's fault when things go wrong; your drinking is never to be blamed. It's out of your control.
- *Drink expects you to stay and be loyal.* It distorts reality and keeps you from seeing things as they really are; what you remember is that alcohol "helped you" get through that difficult moment last time, so you'll stick with it. It holds out "hope" that, if things didn't go well today and you crossed the line, it doesn't matter; tomorrow everything is going to be as you want it to be.
- *Drink is a negative influence on your mental and emotional state.* Under the influence of alcohol, you might have sudden mood swings, from being sweet and funny to angry or rude in a short time.
- *Drink is harmful to your health.* Keeping your drink close to you puts you at risk for increased physical health issues, such as heart problems, cancer, and weight concerns.

The 3Cs: Casual, Central, Committed

Take a look at your relationship with alcohol as parallel to an intimate relationship:
- You may have a *casual relationship* with alcohol if you drink frequently, but alcohol isn't central in your life. Crossing the line would be rare but possible in the long term. Just as a relationship with an acquaintance can grow over time as you see the person more frequently, the same can happen with alcohol; the relationship can move from casual to central. So, think about the consequences when you start drinking more often.

- You may have a *central relationship* with alcohol in which drinking is vital: Alcohol is part of your daily routine and planning. Every occasion is suitable for a drink, and all your social activities revolve around alcohol consumption. Nevertheless, you may not consider that you *already* have an alcohol problem, except for an occasional flash of clarity. As your relationship with alcohol becomes closer, problems arise in your other relationships.
- One more step, and you might be in a *committed relationship* with alcohol. You feel strongly attached to your drink, with signs of substantial psychological and often physical dependence. Being in this kind of relationship will make you drink every day and cross the line consistently. You and booze have moved in, you live together, and all other relationships and realities take second place. This creates a profound change in your life. You may start having difficulties with your job, family, and health, as you become self-absorbed with your drink. Alcohol will turn out to be your primary commitment or priority.

Given continual, consistent drinking over time, your relationship with your lover—alcohol—goes from casual to central, and from central to committed. Take our original quiz in the Appendix to find out whether your relationship with alcohol is casual, central, or committed.

Facing the Obstacles within

Because of how much drinking has become part of ordinary life in our society, you may be in a state of *denial* regarding your relationship with alcohol and disagree or disregard that this lover is problematic. Denial

Introduction

warps your sense of agency so that you feel either powerless to control your drink or *falsely confident that you're in control or can easily regain control*. The societal conditioning you've accepted so far normalizes and glorifies alcohol—this is what's familiar—and you may feel social pressure to continue or increase your drinking.

The idea of change is uncomfortable and therefore seems unnecessary or impossible. Your lover has tricked you into thinking it's easier to maintain the status quo, so you look for evidence to validate thinking that there's no problem with your drinking or, at least, not a significant problem. You believe that life without your lover will be worse; you won't be able to have fun, manage stress, fit in, or be accepted by others. These are *limiting beliefs* that keep you stuck inside your comfort zone with your lover, but because the comfort zone feels known to you and "under control," it feels "good" to stay there.

Limiting beliefs create a *negative mindset* (attitude) toward facing the ups and downs of life, especially the downs. Changing your relationship with alcohol may also come with a risk of loss, whether about how you perceive yourself *("I'm fun and social with alcohol")*, capacity to manage *("I can't unwind or go to sleep without a drink")*, or sense of belonging *("I have to drink to be part of my social circle")*. If we fear loss, our mindset becomes fixed, closed to change. You may be questioning yourself (the *flash of clarity*), but denial, limiting beliefs, a negative mindset, fear of loss, and fear of leaving your comfort zone hold you back from making changes or believing that you can (*loss of self-confidence*). You may look to your lover even more, creating powerful and negative expectations for what alcohol gives you. But leaning on alcohol leaves you numb and powerless, and the more you expect from your drink, the more trapped it leaves you.

When you consistently cross the line, you become an expert in playing the *victim*. Circumstances are out of your hands, and it's not your fault, so *you* don't have to change. It's easy to rationalize crossing the line with alcohol to support a victim mentality. *"Today was such a difficult day, I deserve to drink. I'll drink less tomorrow."*

While you keep drinking, your self-esteem and self-confidence shrink. As your lover moves into the driver's seat, gradually you believe more and more that *you're not good enough on your own,* that you *need* alcohol to manage. These intertwined factors further anchor you to your comfort zone, creating a vicious cycle of crossing the line more and more, limiting your possibilities for positive change. Our program will show you how to leave this seductive but destructive lover.

A Road Map for the Journey Ahead

On the journey ahead, our purpose is to support you in: (1) understanding what keeps you from thinking critically about your relationship with alcohol, (2) becoming empowered to leave your comfort zone with alcohol and move into learning and growth, and (3) living your desired reality as your best self.

We encourage you to look beyond the usual societal acceptance of alcohol, the gender-stereotyped advertising targeting women, and the cultural messages that promote "freedom" and "being yourself." These messages often distract us from the importance of questioning our drinking habits and recognizing the risks of dependency and related issues.

We invite you to reconsider your drinking and, if you dare, to take as many steps on this adventure as you can. Write down what reconsidering your drinking means for you today, and check back with this definition as you go. You might even be inspired to venture toward living alcohol free, once you see the results. The basis of this journey is being curious, thinking critically and personally about alcohol, and taking steps toward living authentically, from your true self—living your best life.

There will be obstacles ahead: the seductive pull of your lover, the coziness of the comfort zone, limiting beliefs, negative mindsets, fear of loss, and the stages of grief,[5] we can experience when ending a relationship and going through change. Trust yourself to hang in there; to keep taking steps, however big or small; to not let fear hold you back.

This is a lover that won't go easily. It's taking so much from you that it wants to remain close and will use all its seductive powers to convince you to keep drinking the same or more. Drink will remind you of the happy times together but minimize the hangovers, interpersonal difficulties, lost sleep, and negative health effects as just "tiny details" in the bigger picture of your relationship.

So, around the midpoint of this journey, we're going to challenge you to a big practical step in reconsidering your drinking: to break up with alcohol for twenty-one days. Whatever your personal big-picture goal in reconsidering alcohol, taking a short break from drinking will help your body to readjust to what's normal for you. If your goal is to moderate your drinking, giving your body a break to lower tolerance will help you to be more successful. If your goal is to be alcohol free, you will be three weeks farther into your journey. *It's up to you!*

We designed this method in order to provide you with practical information and support on transforming beliefs, rewiring mindsets, developing creative new routines and habits, and setting new expectations. We'll walk together through the Learning Zone Model,[6] so that

---

5. Elisabeth Kubler-Ross and David Kessler, *On Grief and Grieving* (Simon and Schuster, 2014).
6. The Learning Zone Model was originally developed by Lev Vygotsky and built upon by Tom Senninger and other psychologists and educators. It presents the framework of the comfort zone, fear zone, learning zone, and growth zones, and how we can move through these zones with preparation, courage, and success to achieve our goals.

you can move from the comfort zone, through the fear zone, and into the learning and growth zones. We'll guide you through the stages of grief, as a framework to identify what you might be feeling and to support integrating change. We'll offer suggestions on how to manage specific social situations and contexts during different parts of the journey (comfort, fear, learning, or growth zones). You'll be well on your way to inhabiting your new, deeper, and more liberated identity, with all the tools you need to maintain your course as you interact with your family, friends, and colleagues, or perhaps with the new tribe you'll gain along the way.

We're excited to venture with you into the extraordinary potential of who you are and all you can do, living life on your own terms.

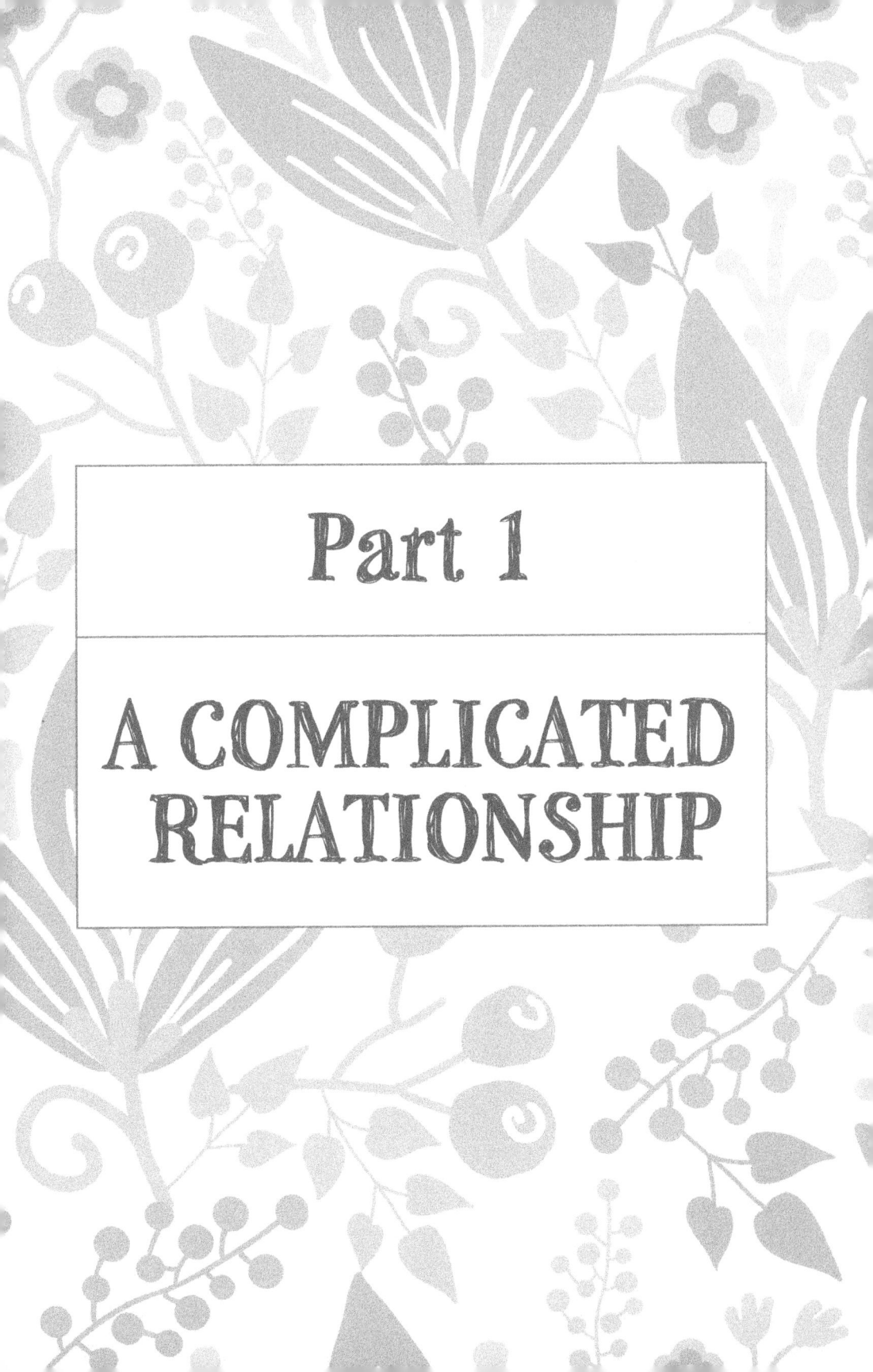
Part 1

A COMPLICATED RELATIONSHIP

CHAPTER 1

WOMEN AND ALCOHOL

In this chapter we discuss the unique ways in which women relate to drinking and how it affects them differently from men, why drinking among women is on the rise, how the COVID-19 pandemic consolidated this trend, and the consequences of alcohol abuse.

We introduce the "feminine drinking culture" and how this affects women's perception and use of alcohol. The appendix includes a quiz that will give you an idea of which one of the 3Cs (Casual, Central, or Committed) you are in your relationship with alcohol.

Historically, men have always consumed more alcohol than women. But studies over the past twenty years show that drinking among women in the United States is on the rise, especially for women ages 38–47.[7,8] These same increases were not shown for men drinkers, meaning that the gender gap in alcohol use is shrinking.

Although women drink less than men in general, women usually experience harsher and more significant effects from alcohol due to

---

7. Aaron White et al., "Converging Patterns of Alcohol Use and Related Outcomes among Females and Males in the United States, 2002 to 2012," *Alcoholism: Clinical and Experimental Research* 39, no. 9 (September 2015):1712–1726. PMID: 26331879.
8. Tim Slade et al., "Birth Cohort Trends in the Global Epidemiology of Alcohol Use and Alcohol-Related Harms in Men and Women: Systematic Review and Metaregression," *BMJ Open* 6, no. 10 (October 24, 2016):e011827, doi: 10.1136/bmjopen-2016-011827.

biological differences in body chemistry and structure. Likely because women typically weigh less and have less total body water as compared to men, the same quantity of alcohol will have a more significant, quicker, and longer-lasting effect on a woman as compared to a man.[9,10]

The consequences of persistent alcohol abuse are also different: Women are more likely than men to develop an alcohol disorder and other alcohol-related health problems, such as cirrhosis or liver damage, high blood pressure, and breast cancer.[11,12,13]

Social and cultural contexts of alcohol consumption have different characteristics across genders. Men drink primarily for positive reinforcement and to share an experience (for instance, meeting friends at a bar and watching a game). Women do the same, but frequently, they drink in relation to problems, pressures, and personal negative states.

Unfortunately, women don't often seek help regarding their alcohol use. Tim Slade and his colleagues at the National Drug and Alcohol Research Centre in Australia write that, "while women seek treatment for almost every other physical and mental health problem at higher rates than men, women who experience problems related to alcohol generally don't seek treatment."[14]

---

9. Aaron M. White, "Gender Differences in the Epidemiology of Alcohol Use and Related Harms in United States," *Alcohol Research Current Reviews* 40, no. 2, accessed May 2023, https://arcr.niaaa.nih.gov/volume/40/2/gender-differences-epidemiology-alcohol-use-and-related-harms-united-states.
10. "Excessive Alcohol Use Is a Risk to Women's Health," *Centers for Disease Control and Prevention (CDC)*, last reviewed October 17, 2022, accessed May 2023, https://www.cdc.gov/alcohol/fact-sheets/womens-health.htm.
11. White, Aaron M. "Gender Differences in the Epidemiology of Alcohol Use and Related Harms in United States," *Alcohol Research Current Reviews* 40, no. 2, accessed May 2023, https://arcr.niaaa.nih.gov/volume/40/2/gender-differences-epidemiology-alcohol-use-and-related-harms-united-states.
12. "Excessive Alcohol Use," *CDC*, last reviewed October 17, 2022.
13. "Women and Alcohol," *National Institute on Alcohol Abuse and Alcoholism (NIAAA)*, updated March 2023, accessed May 2023, https://www.niaaa.nih.gov/publications/brochures-and-fact-sheets/women-and-alcohol.
14. Tim Slade, Cath Chapman, and Maree Teeson, "Women's Alcohol Consumption Catching up to Men: Why This Matters," *National Drug and Alcohol Research Centre*, accessed July 2023, https://ndarc.med.unsw.edu.au/blog/womens-alcohol-consumption-catching-men-why-matters.

Chapter 1: Women and Alcohol

What's behind the Rise in Women's Drinking?

Cultural norms around women's drinking have changed dramatically over the years. The range has varied from drinking certain types of alcohol or drinking in public being considered *taboo*, to women being *legally permitted* to drink in public, to alcohol being *accepted* and having a place in certain social circumstances, to drinking being *usual and expected* in almost any situation, to the point where drinking until inebriated is not considered a problem in some settings. A client recently told us: *"It's okay to be tipsy occasionally. Nobody thinks less of you if you act silly, saying things you don't mean or getting into arguments, because everybody around knows that's not you; it's because of the alcohol."*

Women are exposed to confusing societal messages about drinking. Alcohol consumption is presented as desirable, and ladies who drink are celebrated. There are gendered alcohol products and marketing that target women specifically. Social and other media imply that people need alcohol to cope with their work, family, relationships, and life and that using alcohol in this way is normal—especially for women, given the added emotional and household pressures they experience. Products, movies, online groups, and social structures all contain messages, such as: *"It's your right to drink. Life is better with alcohol."*

Since drinking among women may be related to emotional states or situations, we drink both when we're happy and when we're sad. We drink on weekdays and weekends. We drink during social gatherings and when we're alone; we drink with family and friends; we drink at home, in bars and restaurants, at hair and nail salons. We drink after a long day of work or chores, relaxing over happy hour, at the kids' sports practice, or after the kids have gone to bed. We drink to fit in or at least to try. For most adults who drink, an alcoholic beverage *is considered a good idea in any situation.*

Managing Mood States

Diagnoses of depression and anxiety are on the rise worldwide. Overall, women are more likely to suffer depressive and anxiety disorders. Rising rates of depression and anxiety in women (including due to social pressures) may play a role in the overall increased drinking seen in women.

Alcohol use is often related to negative mood states. Women drink the most when there are troubles or setbacks. In such cases, it's common for women to drink for long hours and to continue drinking until they pass out or go to bed. Drinking is perceived as a way to cope with or regulate mood, but alcohol itself usually intensifies depressive or anxious symptoms, creating a vicious cycle. Imagine the emotional and physical state the next morning—feeling ill, tired, and lacking energy, but with the same problems to manage.

Keeping up with Social Pressures

Social pressures can create or deteriorate emotional negative states. Across cultures, women are bombarded by social expectations. For example:

- Women may be expected to fit in with a particular type of beauty, whether in terms of weight, appearance, fashion, etc.
- Women feel they have to be "perfect" in their personal, social, and professional lives—to "have it all" and be impeccable.
- Many societies still view marriage and motherhood as a woman's destiny with little to no acceptance for even considering other paths.
- Women in unhappy or unhealthy marriages face economic, family, and community pressure to stay with their partners.

- Women may be expected to assume a subordinate role as part of being a "good woman."
- Many women feel pressured to remain silent about sexual harassment.
- Women are considered "natural" caretakers and nurturers, expected to prioritize others' happiness and well-being above their own.
- Ambitious, independent women are viewed with suspicion and may be considered selfish. But a woman who prioritizes family over a career may be judged as "aimless" or "without ambition."

Women are under tremendous pressure to fulfill societal, community, religious, and family ideals. They often feel under scrutiny or blamed for not living up to these unrealistic expectations or for wanting to go a different way. Often, they internalize these feelings, as though they are at fault, which results in shame and guilt: *"I'm not good enough"; "I didn't do my best"; "I should do more."*

Many women use alcohol, whether subconsciously or otherwise, as a way to calm external and internalized pressures. Single mothers, stay-at-home moms, professionals under stress or required to attend company events, shy women, women going through divorces, or empty nesters may feel compelled to drink often, believing that *alcohol helps them to cope with the challenges they face.* Slowly, alcohol becomes a crucial part of their lives and daily routines.

If other women are doing this too, women's social environments become a space to gain validation from other women and find shared rationale or justification for drinking-related behaviors and decisions. *"It's not your fault." "They just don't understand you." "You did the best you could." "You deserve this drink."*

Drinking can make people forget the weight of life's pressures and demands, at least for that evening or social gathering. As the saying goes, *"Alcohol is not the answer, but it makes you forget the question."* Within the context of the feminine drinking culture—women drinking in women-populated social circles—it's easier to find some release and have a relaxing moment.

COVID-19 and Alcohol Consumption among Women

The COVID-19 pandemic and its ongoing aftermath has been one of the most collectively stressful periods in 21st-century history, with countless individual and communal traumas. Connected to an increase in stress, anxiety, and depression during the pandemic, there was also an escalation in women's use of alcohol. A RAND survey study with self-reported data showed that women's days of heavy drinking increased by 41 percent during the pandemic.[15]

Humans need connection, and the pandemic created or increased in-person isolation. Loneliness and lost connections can heighten the risk of depression. Consider that during the pandemic, many people experienced a number of highly stressful events simultaneously in a close period of time, such as the death of a loved one; job loss; loss of opportunities for promotion; loss of a business or livelihood; impossibility of seeing friends or relatives; loss of established routines and pre-COVID life; boredom; loss of hopefulness and things to look forward to, etc.

Anxiety soared due to greater personal and societal uncertainties and emotional stress, whether about finances, layoffs, job issues, rela-

---

15. Michael Pollard, Joan S. Tucker, and Harold D. Green Jr., "Changes in Adult Alcohol Use and Consequences during the COVID-19 Pandemic in the US," *JAMA Network Open* 3, no. 9 (September 29, 2020), doi:10.1001/jamanetworkopen.2020.22942.

tionships, raising a family, and general fear of the unknown future—effects that linger to this day. Many women had to take on additional responsibilities, such as working from home while also caring for and home-schooling their children and taking care of relatives. Relationship and interfamily stresses increased due to everyone being home all the time and lack of space.

As situational factors changed, people started to drink more and in different contexts: at home, alone, anytime. *Since I don't have anywhere to go, what's wrong with having a drink at home? Why not have a drink any time? I don't have to go to the office, or pick up the kids, or drive to sports or activities anyway. I need to find ways to unwind and enjoy something.* We also had more time on our hands, and drinking to fill that time seemed like a good idea. Our relationship with alcohol became more complicated in a short time.

The Feminine Drinking Culture

We talk about alcohol and drinking being part of our culture. Culture includes the beliefs, social norms, and behaviors of a social group. It's the set of shared values, attitudes, drives, and social practices that characterizes a group. Culture defines how groups of people live their lives; it implies *what they know, what they believe, and how they behave.*

In general, people usually accept the various elements of their culture without really thinking much about them. There are two main reasons for this: (1) We learn beliefs, norms, and behaviors from family and people we love, idealize, or imitate. (2) We experience acceptance and integration with our desired group if we follow their specific cultural norms; otherwise, we risk being judged and excluded.

On a big-picture scale, drinking has been practiced in *human cultures* for millennia, as part of social, religious, ritual, celebratory, and healing or medicinal traditions. There are many historical and sociocultural reasons for drinking, and almost all of them can be considered valid or understandable, depending on context. We drink to celebrate, to be part of family and social traditions.

In the US and other countries within its sphere of influence, drinking has become part of our *national culture*. Drinking is a behavior that's accepted and, subsequently, may be expected and anticipated in a variety of settings. In our contemporary culture, people primarily drink to enhance sociability, for personal enjoyment, to escape problems, and to relieve stress.

The social norm that follows is that drinking has become required in almost all social situations involving *women*. What fuels this norm is a belief that alcohol consumption is a positive component of women's lives and interactions.

In the last decade, and mainly in the US, a new kind of feminine identity has started to develop that's related to drinking-centered events and activities, beyond the occasional happy hour or girls' night out. Alcohol is included in almost all situations in which women get together. If there are no drinks, the party or gathering is considered not fun or interesting enough to attend. This has created an additional cultural space where drinking is normalized that is termed the *feminine drinking culture* (FDC).

From our social observations over many years, the feminine drinking culture helps women develop a friendship and a support system and dissipates envy and competition between us. With alcohol, women may feel more outgoing and fun, less inhibited or reserved, and ready to mingle with the group. Conversations usually revolve around personal topics and gossip—dating, kids, family pressures, exercise, health, nutrition, partner's level of attachment, successes or failures at work, etc. In short, alcohol plays a role in female friendships, and women may use alcohol as a tool to enhance socializing, trust, and intimacy.

To be part of the feminine drinking culture, women are conditioned by their social groups to believe:

- Women shouldn't criticize other women for drinking alcohol.
- Women shouldn't be concerned about drinking.
- Drinking is an essential part of personal life and social activities.
- Drinking is *the* way to relax and decompress.
- There are only two types of drinkers: those who can control themselves (us = social or recreational drinkers) and those who can't (them = people who depend on or abuse alcohol).

There are tremendous social pressures in the feminine drinking culture. Even in the context of women's social groups, there is strong peer pressure and mixed messages directed to and internalized by women.[16] On the one hand, there may be pressure not only to drink but also to continue drinking until one becomes tipsy or moderately drunk. At the same time, women consuming alcohol are expected to maintain their "femininity" and "keep it together"—no gross excesses, vomiting, anger, or physical aggression (as men might display). Even tipsiness must be feminine and charming—fun, funny, witty, and relaxed.

What do women get from this drinking culture? First, there's the idea that drinking makes you easygoing and free, helping you to be more spontaneous, to do and say things with less self-censure. This can give you the idea that a better, more fun, and friendly version of you will

---

[16]. Women are often put in a double bind regarding alcohol use and caught between conflicting, opposing messages. On the one hand, "Stand up to gendered taboos and stigma about drinking alcohol; don't worry about it," and on the other hand, "If you drink too much and damage your health or gain weight, it's your fault."

emerge under the influence of alcohol. Second, women drink to feel included and accepted, to not be different from their friends, to be part of the group, to be treated as a member. Third, alcohol can give you space to construct a social identity with the most outgoing parts of yourself and without judgment from others.

With this new social identity, you can connect with other women and accumulate social capital, defined by Granfield and Cloud as "the social relations ... and the resources that potentially flow from these relations."[17] In the feminine drinking culture, alcohol is an essential resource for accelerating social cohesion, expanding social networks, and enabling friendships.

The most important reinforcing aspect of the feminine drinking culture is that while women feel tipsy or "barely drunk," willingness to be vulnerable increases and can lead to developing a strong bond, with confidences and closeness shared that create a sisterhood between the women involved. Loyalties develop; we take care of each other. The problem is that if alcohol is the *main, unifying component* of a group dynamic, the group members will always seek out and include alcohol consumption in order to maintain that same level of connection, reinforcing that dynamic.

In this scenario, drinking moderately or not at all contradicts the normalization and expectation of drinking. Pressure to participate in the feminine drinking culture is linked with belonging and trustworthiness: *"If you don't drink, you don't belong. We can't trust you."* The woman who is reconsidering her drinking or choosing to be alcohol free becomes an outsider, a stranger who can't be trusted. Group members may feel judged by a sober person and are likely to avoid inviting that "miserable sober" woman to the next get-together.

---

17. Robert Granfield and William Cloud, *Coming Clean: Overcoming Addiction without Treatment* (New York: New York University Press, 1999).

Women who want to drink less or take a break from alcohol often feel they have to manage the situation carefully in order to not be rejected or have others conclude that it must be because they have a problem with alcohol. The typical assumptions are that (1) if, you're not an alcoholic, you don't have any reason to quit, and (2) if you stop drinking, you'll miss out on an important component of life and social situations.

Managing this might mean preparing a "good excuse," such as, *"I'm genetically predisposed to alcoholism and can't drink more than one glass,"* or, *"I'm taking one dry month for health reasons or because I need to lose X pounds."* Because women face so much pressure regarding their appearance, "trying to lose weight" or "being on a diet" can be seen as strong explanatory factors for taking a break from alcohol, being sober curious, or alcohol free.

Your friends can make you feel uncomfortable if you choose to drink less or refuse to drink. "Why?" they may question and challenge you, as though something is wrong with you. Their questions and social influence may wear you down over time, making you question your decision or change your mind and revert to your old drinking habits, sabotaging your progress. Some people or groups will do whatever it takes to get you to drink again, because in their minds, you're missing out on all the fun, and they want to "help" you.

Running the risk of being excluded from your usual social group(s), especially if they drink a lot and feel uncomfortable with your change of pace, is a real social pressure that women face. Underlying the feminine drinking culture is the idea that women *should* drink alcohol, that we *need* alcohol to have fun, to enjoy an experience, to feel spirited. If we're anxious in social situations, we may drink (or feel we "should"), because alcohol makes us relax and have more fun. The implicit belief is that people and events are boring and constricted without alcohol. But with alcohol, it's exactly the opposite—anything and everything is possible.

Find out whether you are part of the feminine drinking culture by taking our quiz. (See Appendix.)

"I Can't Imagine Life without Drinking!"

"I can't imagine life being sober. This is a real trap for me. When I awake in the morning, I know that whatever happens, I'll have my wine time in the evening. A bad day at the office? An argument with my partner? A problem with my son? I'll forget all of these in the evening! More than forgetting, it's that I won't think about those issues anymore for today, and I won't care about them until tomorrow.

"In my circle, drinking is part of daily routines and events, both at home and out with friends. If you don't drink, you're not part of our group, or we think you might have been an alcoholic before or that you have a drinking problem. If I take a break from alcohol, I'll be changed into somebody I don't like—less chatty and outgoing—and I'll feel like an outsider in my social circle.

"Another reality that holds me back from giving up alcohol is that I can't imagine being on vacation or celebrating and having water or Diet Coke when everybody else is drinking fabulous champagne." —Martha

When alcohol is involved in every part of life, imagining how we could ever stay sober (or soberish) is a significant obstacle in making a change. *How will I get through everyday pressures? How will I maintain my friendships when most of my circle drink?* And an important one related to our sense of self: *Without alcohol, my personality will change. I won't be outgoing, fun, and calm. I'll be that boring person nobody wants to hang out with.*

This trap has a rock-solid foundation: *We feel we need alcohol to have a good time, to be good enough, or to be accepted.* But staying with this status quo, not making any changes, will *always* lead to negative consequences.

The only way out of this trap is to reframe our foundation: Happy times and feeling good are *not* because of the effects of alcohol. They can be connected to interactions with friends, progress or success, the shared joy or relief of an occasion or moment (a celebration; the time of the day when we're finished with obligations). Feeling more outgoing or being freer when we drink is on us; we can experience those effects through other means. They can be based on our authentic resources, not on the short-term, misleading effects of alcohol. We assure you that you can have joy, fun, camaraderie, and relaxation that doesn't depend on alcohol.

To get started on overcoming this trap, we must change our outlook: Think about something you may have been addicted to in the past and feel differently about now. For example, if you smoked in the past, you probably remember that it was a strong habit and extremely challenging to quit. But you did it, and now you can't imagine smoking again—even the smell of cigarettes might make you sick.

Booze is the same. Staying with the habit of alcohol will make your life harder than it needs to be. *Why not make a choice that prioritizes your well-being?* Drinking moderately or quitting will benefit you by reestablishing your mental, relational, spiritual, economic, and health equilibrium. You can find happiness and excitement with a lifestyle that doesn't require alcohol. We have only one shot at this life, and you must decide how to make it truly count.

See drinking for what it is: a habit that keeps you trapped inside a small space of limited possibility. It doesn't let you see your reality and self clearly. It causes your mental and physical health to suffer and puts your relationships under stress. Take control of this area of your life by reducing the risk of harmful effects of drinking. Without the invalidating effects of alcohol, you will be better able to reconnect with yourself, to be present, and to live an authentic life. You will feel more than good enough!

Say it with us: *Life without alcohol will be wonderful, and I will no longer be controlled by alcohol or suffer the negative consequences of drinking.* You've got this!

Quiz: What's Your Relationship with Alcohol?

What kind of relationship are you actually in with alcohol? Find out whether your relationship with alcohol is casual, central, or committed by taking our quiz. (See Appendix.)

Notes:

CHAPTER 2
CROSSING THE LINE

Crossing the line doesn't mean that you have an alcohol disorder or are an "alcoholic," but it's a sign that alcohol has become a habit that's part of most of your social activities, an organizing factor in your life, and keeps taking up space. Here are some practical signs that might indicate you're crossing the line with alcohol:

- Your tolerance for alcohol has increased so you drink more to gain the same effects.
- You drink more than you've planned. Say that yesterday you had two or three drinks more than usual, so your plan today is to stay within your limits or not drink at all. However, you drink again, and maybe more than regularly.
- People who care about you and are close to you—a friend, partner, or parent—express concerns. They worry about how much or how often you drink and how dependent you've become on alcohol.
- You drink by yourself in addition to drinking at social events.
- You have regrets about how much you drink.
- You repeatedly have hangovers—a clear signal that something must change.

- You don't remember conversations or things that happened recently due to alcohol intake.
- You don't sleep well, or you wake up in the night once the initial effects of alcohol drop off.
- You look forward to drinking as something to cheer you up, relieve an unpleasant mood, or mitigate your boredom.
- You need a drink before, during, or after joyful, stressful, or sad situations. Alcohol is the partner that helps you get through any circumstance.
- Your life is structured around drinking, whether at home (how much booze you have, if you must buy more and when), or at parties or various gatherings (making sure that the places you go to are serving the type of alcohol you like).
- Those times that you *need* a drink and crave alcohol and can't stop obsessing about this are becoming more frequent. You think about your drinking as something *significant and ever-present* in your life.
- You may get upset when someone points out how much you are drinking.
- You may hide, reduce, or avoid disclosing how many drinks you normally have.

Whether any of these examples of crossing the line with alcohol have come up for you, maybe you don't think of your drinking as a problem in your everyday life. But it's possible you've had the flash of clarity that makes you wonder about your drinking, hangovers, routines, health, or weight. You're starting to think about whether your relationship with alcohol takes more than it gives you. You may worry about what will happen in your immediate and distant future if you stay on this path: *Will you develop a disorder or dependency? Will your health be affected? Will you gain weight? Will your children, partner, or family suffer because of your choices?*

Maybe you face a dilemma. What would be worse: To quit alcohol and possibly lose the feelings of fun and acceptance you have when you drink? Or to risk continuing a habit that will become stronger, with more negative outcomes, over time?

In this chapter we'll explain more about the elements of crossing the line in relation to the normalization of drinking; the denial associated with the place alcohol has in our society; the excitement of anticipating a drink (or a few); the flash of clarity; the day after, experiencing hangovers more often; and the power of shame, anger, guilt, and self-loathing.

The Normalization of Drinking

"I'm a wife and a mother, and everything in my life looks fine, but I've had a secret for a long time: I'm drinking too much. I had my daughter a couple years ago. I was in a new city, without friends or family. I started attending the moms' group in my neighborhood. Each of us brought a bottle of wine for the get-together, and by the end of the night, there was no wine left—we drank it all. I started to like this, drinking with my new friends.

"My husband travels for work nearly every week and then hangs out with his own friends. I'm by myself with my daughter most of the time. I started buying wine to drink after she'd gone to sleep. Now it's a habit to drink every day. Some friends showed me how to mix vodka with Gatorade, so I could carry a bottle in my purse everywhere. Drinking is

part of my daily routine, and it's important to me. This isn't wrong, in my opinion, and my friends think so, too. On the contrary, it helps to relieve the stress, exhaustion, and solitude of basically parenting alone. It's fun and it's fine, as long as I can manage my daily life.

"My husband has been surprised sometimes and tells me, 'Take it easy.' He doesn't understand that drinking is totally okay if you can control how much you drink, if you aren't getting drunk, passing out, or blacking out every night. It's become a point of friction between us." —Celine

Normalization refers to the way in which ideas, attitudes, or behaviors come to be seen as "normal," "acceptable," and part of cultural norms and regular routines. This can happen with ideas or practices that were considered wrong or inappropriate previously and now are deemed appropriate and correct. If an activity or behavior is considered "what's right," we can more easily agree with and accept it, because it's not in conflict with social norms about how to live or conduct ourselves.

Let's return to the feminine drinking culture that influences our minds and feelings to accept that not only is drinking okay but it's also:

- A *right* that we've earned as adult women.
- A *need*, given all the extra labor and pressures women have to manage.
- *What everybody does.* Why should we be excluded from normal, fun, relaxing activities by ourselves or with our social circles? If we don't drink, we run the risk of missing out or feeling like we don't belong.

Alcohol use has become so normalized that behaviors like sobriety or reduced drinking have become unusual, even something to be avoided or feared. In many social circles, people say that only those with a serious drinking problem should reduce their drinking or practice sobriety; the rest of us don't need to, because we have it under control. The truth is that we don't. Alcohol is an addictive substance; it's only a matter of time until it controls us.

The normalization of drinking not only covers moderate, regular alcohol use but also extends to binge drinking or heavy alcohol consumption. In certain situations, taking drinking to this extreme is even encouraged. One client told us, *"If you're at a wedding and you're staying at the venue for the night, what's wrong with drinking until you pass out? You don't have to drive back home, everyone is drinking a lot, and nobody expects anything from you."*

As part of the normalization of drinking, you might have said or heard these types of comments:

- *"Everyone drank a lot last night, so I had no choice."*
- *"It's New Year's Eve. Of course, I'm going to drink until I feel tipsy or drunk."*
- *"I met my friends at a bar and had a couple glasses of wine. We continued talking and ordering drinks to our table, and I realized we'd all had at least four drinks each in a short time."*
- *"After a long and stressful day, a drink or two is what I need. Sometimes I keep drinking until I go to bed."*

Read that list again, and see what sort of reactions these comments bring up for you and how they land. These comments are also examples of crossing the line.

Within the feminine drinking culture, the normalization of drinking implies that most women-oriented activities will include alcohol as an essential component of the gathering. Even baby showers or kids' birthdays will include wine, champagne, mimosas, or other drinks. Sometimes the alcohol being served is *the* reason to show up. Events that don't include drinking are considered boring and not worth attending.

Anticipation

Anticipation is looking forward to something, usually pleasurable or exciting, that you expect to happen. Anticipation is part of the fun, good times, or happiness that we hope or expect the actual experience will give us.

When it comes to drinking, anticipation typically focuses on the *desirable, tempting aspects*—real or perceived—of alcohol use: a sense of fun, cutting loose, being with family or friends, feeling relaxed, enjoyable tastes, and so on. But there's an *idealization* that comes with this anticipation that makes you see the "positive" and enjoyable parts of drinking only. You don't anticipate the conflicting, harmful, or problematic aspects of alcohol. You don't remember the hard fight you sometimes have with yourself to not cross the line, or the negative feelings and consequences that come from drinking in excess. In idealized anticipation, only the good and attractive expectations count; the rest—and certainly anything negative—doesn't exist.

Anticipation is the first part of a vicious cycle with alcohol. People usually do experience some positives with drinks one or two, which reinforces the positive anticipation and idealization of alcohol. But following closely behind are all the negatives that pile up as you keep drinking: over-imbibing; feeling sick; remorse and self-questioning; complete disregard for the unpleasant parts of the episode; and finally, feeling ready to start all over. Anticipation kicks in again.

If you've experienced this cycle and are being realistic, you can see that you're giving drinking more time, energy, and money than you should.

If you're focused only on the "positives" of drinking and you consider the negatives to be temporary, brief, and linked to specific situational factors—but *not to the drinking*—then your thinking isn't objective.

Maybe your justification is that the people you're with are drinking heavily, too. You hang out with the same group often and drink more than you want, because these people are part of your comfort zone; or you may drink more because of the events you're attending. In any case, drinking the amount you do is *never your fault*. It's always about *other* people or circumstances, and you use these factors to justify or excuse your choices.

> *"I grew up in a drinking culture, and I couldn't question the routines surrounding alcohol. Fridays to Sundays was 'party time,' when drinking was unlimited. You just had to 'understand how to drink.' Life looks great in this culture; drinking times are full of fun and social interactions.*
>
> *"After going through so many of these weekends, I learned that what I was doing was pretty bad for me. I always imagined myself as being fun, witty, cool, and having enjoyable moments with my friends. The reality was that after the first two to three drinks, I couldn't manage what happened next. My hangovers became more frequent and lasted longer and I felt bad about myself and my choices. Nothing happy at all.*
>
> *"At first I blamed the situation and the people I was with. But then I realized that I was the one idealizing alcohol. What I was looking forward to wasn't actually real. How can a moment be perfect when you and everyone else there aren't at 100 percent? I realized that I could actually ruin my life if I ignored the fallacies of this 'anticipation.' Why drink alcohol to have fun when we know that alcohol has ruined millions of lives? My life could be the next one, if I don't change."* —Theresa

The idea that drinking is what allows you to have happiness and fun is a myth. The opposite is true: Alcohol makes you feel numb and low energy but quick to react in a negative way. It lowers inhibition and self-control, making you act differently from when you're sober. The personality you get when you're drinking is not you.—*Not the real you.*

There are two reasons for being cautious about the anticipatory effects of drinking. The first is that it could hide that you might be crossing the line and developing an addiction to alcohol. Anticipation may lead you to expect that alcohol will enhance your experiences. In reality, with time, alcohol will distort your experiences and ruin your health, relationships, income, and overall life—and in the meantime, your habit of drinking has become only stronger.

The second is when anticipation gets mixed up with expectation.[18] In some cases, expectation can be a positive element, because it provides direction and excitement to go forward. But expectations can also be unrealistic and cause stress, disappointment, and self-depreciation. The most important element in relation to drinking is that expectations can be rigid. We have a single outcome in mind *("Drinking makes me fun!" "I have a good time with alcohol!" "Drinking is how I'm part of this group."),* and we try to hold ourselves to it to make our predictions happen. If reality doesn't go according to our pre-set expectations, disappointment and annoyance set in quickly.

To counter alcohol-related expectations, you could start cultivating a healthy and realistic sense of anticipation for other positive activities and routines that don't rely on or include drinking, like going for a walk, hiking, a yoga or fitness class, meeting a new group, exploring places, taking up a sport or hobby. You can redirect the feelings and anticipation linked with drinking to other healthier activities and routines that truly reward your sense of anticipation with fun and enjoyment.

---

18. What's the difference between anticipation and expectation? Anticipation is when you feel and know something is coming up and you're hoping for it to happen. Expectation is what you consider is going to happen but is not guaranteed. For example: "My anticipation for this party is killing me!" "My expectations for this party are good."

Chapter 2: Crossing the Line

The Flash of Clarity

The flash of clarity is a type of moment of truth. When it comes to alcohol use, it can feel like a sudden realization that *something is wrong, something is outside our control, we'll face unwanted consequences if we don't change.*

A flash of clarity is like an *awakening*, an unexpected self-awareness related to how much or how frequently we drink; how intensely we anticipate having a drink; how bad our hangovers are; how much money our happy hours cost us. The flash of clarity could also come in relation to more serious issues, like a problem with a friend or a family member, an argument with our partner, a DWI (driving while intoxicated or impaired), or a health problem.

> *"I used to justify my drinking for different reasons, like having problems with my kids, work stress, or arguments with my husband. Day after day, something happened, and I 'needed' or 'deserved' a drink. Until one day, driving to pick up my kids, I had that moment of clarity: drinking is not because of this or that; it's because of me. I should be in control, but I'm not controlling my drinking, and it's becoming worse with time. Will I turn out to be an alcoholic if I continue drinking like this?"* —Glenna

The flash of clarity appears at a point where denial, as a coping or protective mechanism, isn't working for some reason. It's important to pay attention to your flash of clarity; it's a *powerful sign*, a gift. If you don't take any action, eventually the denial will return, justifying your excessive drinking for one reason or another.

A flash of clarity shows us a reality that's unhealthy and could lead to bad consequences and paying high costs in the future. It may feel uncomfortable, but it's a positive factor. A flash of clarity can be the starting point for reconsidering our drinking and beginning our journey of self-reclamation and recovery. It can be the place where we realize that our brakes are failing, and we're going downhill—but that we still have the power to make a change before the fall becomes *uncontrollable.*

This is also where other people can have a decisive influence. The best way to use a flash of clarity is to seek help from those who know how to help you. It could be a friend, family member, or professional—someone who knows you and can help you to realign and regain control, so you can live life the way you want to, free from negative patterns.

In general, asking for help from someone in your drinking circle may cause you to lose precious time. People from that circle are likely to try to reestablish your denial and make you return to your questioned habit. In fact, it may be essential that you distance yourself from the people with whom you used to drink. They might be struggling with crossing the line themselves and trying to shut down their own internal voice and flash of clarity. If they can't help themselves in this area, they may not be able to help you.

The flash of clarity can appear at any time, especially during or after occasions when you're crossing the line with alcohol. (See the list at the beginning of this chapter for examples.) The flash of clarity might also appear when:

- You realize how much money you're spending on alcohol (never mind on related exceptional expenses, like a DWI, an accident, or hospital bill). Start by looking at how much you're spending at home or when you go out when you order drinks.
- You can't drink and have strong cravings for alcohol. Those times that you *need* a drink and it's all you can think about are becoming more frequent.

- You're not sure if what you said or did was appropriate or could damage meaningful relationships.
- You're not totally in control and clear about your words and actions.

Go ahead and face your flash of clarity. It's powerful and wise. Take it as a gift. Use it to make changes. If nothing changes, eventually you will find yourself in that degrading state where you're no longer totally conscious of your emotions, thoughts, or reactions. Slowly, alcohol will take everything away from you, and you may not even realize it until you get to the point where a rehab program may be the only solution.

The next time you have a flash of clarity, write it down (on your phone, in a notebook, etc.) along with the thoughts, feelings, and questions it brings up. Put this somewhere visible, and read what you wrote every night before going to bed, as soon as you wake up every morning and next time you're tempted to cross the line.

Make a list of all the potential future consequences if you keep drinking like this: the ways in which it could harm you, your relationship with your partner, your kids, your job, your health, your self-esteem, your confidence, your appearance, your weight, your skin, and so on.

Be honest with yourself about what you get and what gets taken from you when you drink. Is it worth it?

What's one thing you can do today to change your future based on what you see now from this powerful place of clarity? Can you replace your drinking patterns with a new habit, routine, activity, or nonalcoholic beverage? *Honor this moment by making a change.* **Now is the time.**

Denial

What does every woman crossing the line hope for? That one day, magically, she'll be able to drink in a controlled way, enjoying the moment and having total command over her decision to continue drinking or not. The persistence of this magical thinking is impressive; it's based on the *denial* that every person uses when crossing the line.

Since we live in a society where alcohol is seen as a positive element in our personal and social lives, we might say, *how can having a little more of something positive be a bad thing?* Besides, according to those who frequently drink in excess, there are two kinds of people, alcoholics and nonalcoholics, and these groups are fundamentally different. People who are alcoholics have a real problem: They can't control how much they drink. Nonalcoholics consider themselves to be capable of restraint: If they overdrink, it's occasional, and not in any way linked to a permanent loss of control.

What causes "nonalcoholics" to cross the line? It's always about something not related to "being an alcoholic," such as any or all of the following:

- Reaction to solitude or boredom (internal discomfort).
- Reaction to overwhelm or social pressures (too much to manage or do).
- Need to belong to a group.
- Need to portray a certain emotional or social state (to be cool, fun, outgoing, etc.).
- Need to have an exciting moment.
- Desire to "escape" reality.
- Desire to end each day "well" and "relaxed," without having to think about what did or didn't happen.
- Parties, holidays, celebrations, events.

Whatever the reason, it's never because *"we"* suffer the lack of control that characterizes *"them"*—people who abuse, or are dependent on, alcohol. When we drink in excess often, we blame internal or external situations and circumstances; drinking is just a consequence of *those* conditions. We humans are very good at self-deception. However, we also have the option to replace this denial with awareness.

So, let's talk about denial. In broad terms, denial is a coping mechanism that we use to try to protect ourselves from surrounding threats (actual or perceived) and to give us time to adapt or respond to complex and new situations. Humans have a tremendous capacity for adaptation, but we need time and an open mind to change.

Denial can be a positive mechanism, especially in the short term, when it's functional. It can allow you to focus on other thoughts or activities without being overwhelmed by a problem; it can give you space to evaluate an issue. Denial can have negative effects when you let it keep you in the dark. Staying in denial can restrict or inhibit our ability to confront problems.

In the case of drinking, denial can "protect you" from recognizing how much you rely on alcohol to manage internal and external factors, and that you've lost control of your alcohol intake. You may think you're in control, *"I can stop anytime!"* But after a while, given the addictive characteristic of alcohol, sooner or later, that control you think you have is no longer a reality.

Maybe you can recognize times when you've lost control and crossed the line. But we usually deny how serious this is. We make an erroneous evaluation of the issue *("It was only one time")* and an overly optimistic evaluation of the future *("I'll drink way less next time")*. The fact is that if you drink in excess on a regular basis, you're entering dangerous territory. The capacity of your control comes and goes and becomes inefficient.

It's vulnerable to realize something is not under your control. Vulnerability means increased discomfort. To avoid or manage these feelings of discomfort, your drinking can escalate in frequency and intensity, with possibly destructive long-term consequences.

In conclusion, denial is only a temporary tactic. When it's used for too long or too often, it keeps you stuck in a vicious cycle that can lead you into a dangerous zone. You need to be *honest and realistic with yourself* (and by getting external help, if needed) to examine the situation and recover your control, *rather than try to justify overdrinking or pretend everything is fine.* If you keep crossing the line over and over, you're not doing okay. End of story.

What helps our clients to move away from denial is to imagine the negative outcomes of not taking action. Let's say you keep drinking like this and crossing the line often; how much is alcohol taking from you? If you continue on this path, what will your life, health, career, finances, and family look like in one, five, or ten years from now?

The Morning After

Carol is fifty-two, married to a lawyer, with twin sons in college—a recent empty nester.

Once Carol's children left for college, she realized that she no longer had much in common with her husband. They had focused so much on raising the twins and forging their careers without investing enough time in their relationship and individual selves. Carol does have more time for social activities now that her boys are away. She has several friends in the neighborhood and is part of a couples' group with her husband, as one of the few things they still do together.

Carol began drinking alcohol a few years before her children moved out. She felt she had a good handle on it when the family was at home together. There were evening routines to attend to that also filled up her time. But once the twins left, she started to drink more. She was more argumentative and easily irritated with her husband. In the mornings, she couldn't give her job her attention. She was often worried about what she may have said or done the night before, as she couldn't remember important details. She didn't feel well physically and emotionally. She was tired all the time.

As her relationship with her husband deteriorated further, she went out more often with friends. Heavy drinking became an almost daily routine. Disagreements with friends and acquaintances were added to the already existing marital discord. She began having difficulties at work, including being late, unprepared for meetings, and making multiple errors in tasks she had practiced for years.

When it comes to crossing the line, "the morning after" can include any of the following:

- Being hungover.
- Becoming conscious of the misadventures of the night before. For instance, personal and relational problems, arguments, health issues, even economic and legal consequences (think of a DWI!). As you gain awareness or hear stories from others, maybe you start thinking that you should never drink again, or you may plan to drink less—intentions that will likely fail the next time you're around alcohol.
- If you can't remember what happened the night before, you're unable to evaluate the seriousness of the problem and the possibility of resolving it. You may feel ashamed and regret whatever happened, but it's embarrassing to acknowledge this, and denial

"protects you" from looking at this uncomfortable part of yourself. At the same time, your confidence is affected, because you couldn't control yourself, and there's nothing that you can do now to fix the past.

We're only human, of course, and it's natural to slip up here and there. Even when we're fine and sober, we can make mistakes and create problems without realizing it. Imagine, though, the complications we can trigger in our personal and social lives when we aren't totally conscious of what we're doing, and our impulsivity is charging ahead on all fronts! When you add in that almost everybody else is under the influence of alcohol, too, the potential for misunderstandings and problems is exponential. Even what seemed excellent or brilliant the night before doesn't look as good in the light of the next day.

Putting it all together: In the morning after, you're feeling unwell physically because of the hangover. This can impact your health, personal and social relationships, and effectiveness at work—all of which can alter your quality of life. You may have doubts and questions about your behavior, which you don't remember well or at all. You may be embarrassed about what you said or did, with potential impacts to your social life and self-confidence. Crossing the line isn't an excuse; whatever has happened doesn't just disappear the following day—all the more so if the events included inappropriate behavior or lead to legal or other serious consequences.

During the morning after, you may have a flash of clarity. Ask yourself: *Is my drinking becoming a problem? Is this what I want in life? What will my life be in one, two, or five years if I continue drinking this way? Should I moderate my drinking or quit altogether?* Listen and respond to your questions. This flash of clarity could be the first step in considering your drinking as a problem that needs your intentional effort to reach a solution.

Use and Honor Past Hangovers

If you haven't experienced a hangover yet, you will if you continue crossing the line. A typical hangover can include some or all of the following symptoms: fatigue, weakness, headache, muscle aches, nausea, stomach pain, sweating, increased blood pressure, and sensibility to light and sound. Your sleep may be disrupted, and when you do wake up, you experience physical discomfort and uneasiness. That can be difficult enough, but in addition, you may also feel anxiety, worry, or embarrassment related to remembering or not remembering what you said or did the night before.

Jackie is a divorced woman in her mid-forties, with a stable university job. When her husband began divorce proceedings, she started to drink more, especially during evenings with her girlfriends. She found some comfort in their conversations, especially when sharing personal information and receiving their support about what she was facing.

> *"I wanted to get through and be done with my divorce in the best way I could, which was a difficult objective, because it was a really nasty divorce. I also wanted to figure out how to redo my life in the only way I could conceive of it at the time—with a partner, not alone. I was insecure about my weight and my face was showing signs of aging. All of this significantly contributed to my worry that I would never get married again."* —Jackie

Jackie was making decisions from a place of loneliness and fear. Her nights out became the only time she felt free of her worries. She began to anticipate feeling this release and expected this effect from drinking but soon realized that she needed more drinks every time to feel worry-free. With increased drinking, she felt hungover the next day, and it affected her work. She lacked energy and made more mistakes. One evening, on the way home from a happy hour, she got a DWI for going just over the speed limit when she thought she was driving normally.

Even after this, she was still indifferent to all these clues—the DWI, poor performance at work, several hangovers per month—because she didn't think she wanted to change. Alcohol was supposedly helping her to cope with the stress and pressure. Every night she felt she had to drink, no matter what, instead of facing and working through her problems. In fact, she didn't think she had a choice other than alcohol. On many of the following mornings, she felt ashamed, thinking about what she'd said the night before and how embarrassed she was.

Think about it...

Maybe your situation isn't as complex as Jackie's, but think about your drinking, and respond to the following questions:

1. What hangover symptoms or feelings have you had (e.g., fatigue, weakness, headache, muscle aches, nausea, stomach pain, sweating, increased blood pressure, and sensibility to light and sound; anxiety, worry, or embarrassment related to remembering or not remembering what you said or did the night before)?
2. How many times a week do you have a hangover?
3. How do you feel the following morning? What's on your mind?
4. Do you make any plans to restrict your drinking when you feel like that?

5. How do you recover from a hangover?
6. Why do you keep allowing yourself to feel like that? What needs to happen for you to make a change?
7. What problems have, or could have, happened when you were drinking or afterward?
8. What consequences could you face soon if you keep drinking like this?

In conclusion, if you've had problems like Jackie, you know what we're talking about. And if you don't know yet, it's just a matter of time. It might take one, five, or fifteen years, but make no mistake, you will have problems if you don't reconsider your drinking. We may start with moments that seem funny or entertaining and end up in serious situations. What we do or say while drinking doesn't disappear when we sober up. And we may not be clear about the severity of what we did or said, which may have consequences and affect future actions.

If all of this isn't enough, remember how bad it feels when you're physically impaired. Do you want to experience any of those unpleasant symptoms again? Alcohol-provoked downfalls happen in real life to all kinds of people. You don't have to be one of them! You still have a choice today, but eventually, alcohol will control you, and the way out will be tougher. *Use and honor your past hangovers by not repeating what caused them.*

Shame, Guilt, and Self-Loathing

Shame

Crossing the line in drinking is closely related to experiencing shame. *Shame* makes us look at our whole self, not just one part, in a negative way. We feel inferior, like a failure; we experience self-loathing.

Shame is different from *guilt*, which is a feeling related to a particular error. Shame is associated with our self-image of our flaws; we believe that they're *intrinsic to who we are*, and we think others perceive us in the same way.

"I'm going to tell you something about myself that I've felt ashamed of for a long time. I don't talk about this with others. It's about my use of alcohol. I drink more than what my family or friends see. I drink on my own before and after I drink with others. I have a shot of whiskey before I go out to feel more outgoing. When I get home, I drink more to relax, unwind, and forget my concerns.

"I worry about other people discovering this about me, because they would see immediately that I can't control myself and that I really need help. I would be ashamed if my family, friends or coworkers were to think that I'm an alcoholic. I want to be happy, but deep inside, I feel sad all the time. I'm a failure. I think I can get my drinking under control before others see how much I drink. But being ashamed makes me feel stuck, with no confidence or possibility to change things. Consequently, I keep drinking the same as before." —Stephanie

In Stephanie's story, we can see the invalidating influence of shame when we drink more than we want. Shame establishes a profound separation between yourself and others. *Internally*, your self-esteem and confidence may be too low to make changes. *Externally*, there's denial and secrecy, which prevents others from knowing the situation and offering help.

Bringing our secrets into the light, practicing self-compassion instead of judgment, and not overidentifying with thoughts and feelings are positive ways to address and overcome shame.

Shame can become anger and blame

Some research makes a connection between shame and anger. We know that people who experience shame direct their hostility toward themselves primarily. In some cases, the experience of shame leaves the person feeling so disgusted that they redirect that hostility outward and blame other people and situations. This is a way to disperse the anger they feel.[19,20] In this case, anger is masking other emotions, such as embarrassment, remorse, or self-doubt.

As you can see, the shift from shame to anger can be a self-defense mechanism. When we repress painful emotions, such as shame, anger can be a way to unleash those contained and constrained feelings, redirecting them to others and "protecting" ourselves from feeling and dealing with them.

People usually cope with shame around alcohol use in two different ways:

1. *Withdrawing*, avoiding exposing our shameful self to others. This isolation creates an illusion of a safe environment, in which we usually tend to drink more and by ourselves.
2. *Blaming and directing anger toward others*, trying to preserve our personal self. Anger grows as we drink—we don't want to say that nasty thing, but the words come out of our mouth anyway. We realize we can't take back what we said, and we feel more shame and regret.

---

19. Jeffrey Stuewig et al., "Shaming, Blaming, and Maiming: Functional Links among the Moral Emotions, Externalization of Blame, and Aggression," *Journal of Research in Personality* 44, no. 1 (February 1, 2010): 91–102. doi: 10.1016/j.jrp.2009.12.005. PMID: 20369025; PMCID: PMC2848360.
20. Suzanne M. Retzinger, "Resentment and Laughter: Video Studies of the Shame-Rage Spiral," in *The Role of Shame in Symptom Formation*, ed. Helen B. Lewis (Hillsdale, NJ: Erlbaum, 1987): 151–181.

Regarding this second way of coping with shame, we should consider that anger is an active emotion of strength, power, and command. By redirecting the feeling of shame to hostility, the self (previously undermined) is re-energized and boosted. Here is Kathy's story:

"I started crossing the line when my child was two years old. I'm a stay-at-home mom, and that gave me the freedom to drink during the day. It was a difficult time for me and my marriage. My relationship with my husband was not very good, and I felt disconnected from him. I had gained some extra pounds that I couldn't lose.

"When I think of myself back then, I can see I wasn't happy, I didn't have any confidence. My drinking began in gatherings with other moms, but after a short time, I also started drinking by myself, and that gave me a comfortable space where I didn't think too much.

"Getting together and drinking with other moms was okay initially, but then our conversations became more gossipy and negative. It didn't pay to be vulnerable with them. I felt they were going to judge me if I didn't show some strength. I wanted to be respected, so it was impossible for me to talk with them about my developing problem with alcohol and to ask for help. I was ashamed about drinking way too much.

"So I also gossiped and pointed out the shortcomings and mistakes of others in the group. That made me feel better about myself because I wasn't the only one with problems. I didn't feel ashamed and mortified about myself, because I perceived the same issues in many of them. I liked what I was doing: drawing attention to their mistakes instead of to my own drinking behavior and relationship problems." —Kathy

Kathy redirected her feelings of shame, turning it into hostility toward others—undermining and judging them, which gave her sense of self a boost.

When we direct our shame outward, who or what do we blame? Everything and everyone else are perfect targets for blame: Our partner, parents, siblings, friends, children, children's teachers, bosses, coworkers, money, overwhelming routines, even the weather. No one and nothing are off limits.—Except for *two things*. Can you guess what they are? That's right: *Your drinking, and yourself!*

Guilt

Guilt is a consequence of an error or mistake we made. In general, most of the mistakes people feel guilty about aren't made with intention of wrongdoing. Nevertheless, *feeling guilty is a familiar sensation to every woman in our culture.* We've been raised and educated with the concept that if we become aware of our wrongdoings and correct them, we ask forgiveness, we learn, we try to make things right, and we become better as a result.

Learning and recognizing that we can do better in the future can be a positive outcome of feeling guilty. But we don't always take this path. The negative side of guilt is unreasonable self-blame and the pervading sense of judgment we direct toward ourselves or others, or that others direct to us.

Sometimes, feeling guilt is understandable, such as when a person knows something is wrong, has the freedom to act or choose differently, but goes ahead and does that thing anyway. When it comes to alcohol, however, given the normalization of drinking in our culture, it's okay to drink, and drinking is considered a positive activity. You have freedom to act differently, but *why not have a drink?* Alcohol is expected, accepted, and legal, so we can drink without guilt. Besides, you or your peers might believe that you've earned a drink, you deserve it, given what you're going through. Other things or people are to blame—your partner, your deadlines, your work, your family, or money—*but not you.*

So, apart from circumstances in which we have clearly behaved poorly toward others, the guilt is usually very personal, *directed from us to ourselves.* You may look at yourself negatively for what you did or said while under the influence, even if no one else says anything to you about it. But a bit of denial may creep in: You may rationalize that the guilt is relative, because you weren't in absolute control of your behavior, so, is it really your fault?

In the case of crossing the line with drinking, it can be difficult to accept responsibility and make amends. The possible responsibility is blurred because of the place that alcohol has in our society where drinking is implicitly okay.

There is a point where *guilt meets shame*. In drinking, we're doing something that pretty much everybody else does and considers fine. But, as it turns out, it's bad for us, and losing control is our responsibility.

Self-Loathing

Self-loathing is very much related to shame and refers to an *extreme criticism of oneself*. It's connected to negative emotional states and can include *constantly* feeling like you aren't good enough, you're worthless, you don't fit in, or you're incapable of doing good things. There may be self-deprecating thoughts and selected memories and stories that reinforce those thoughts.

Self-loathing tends to lead to isolation. We might blame and berate ourselves for things beyond our control. There may be self-directed anger and hatred. It's like bullying yourself.

Low self-esteem can keep us stuck in the same behaviors, even when we think they're bad for us. We can become complacent and familiar with our comfort zone, and low self-esteem may prevent us from making changes to improve our lives.

Building self-esteem is part of the solution to overcoming self-loathing ("I'm weak," "I'm worthless"). *Self-esteem is the motor of the self.* Essentially, it relates to how a person views and values herself, and as a result, it's connected to how much we can trust in and count on ourselves, our resources and potential. Cultivating self-esteem is essential to making changes and progressing.

In conclusion, emotions of shame, guilt, self-loathing, and anger are all connected in relation to drinking and affect people's self-esteem and confidence along with all their possibilities. And, of course, these same feelings contribute to the vicious cycle that keeps us stuck in our drinking routines and can lead us to drink more.

Notes:

CHAPTER 3

WHAT HAPPENS WHEN YOU CROSS THE LINE

By now, you're aware that alcohol is an addictive substance that creates dangerous repercussions that only escalate with time and use. Even if you've thought that you could control things, you recognize that, if you continue with the booze, there's a real possibility you might experience negative consequences.

Our method focuses on taking care of yourself *before* you develop an alcohol disorder, and if you're reading this book, you hopefully haven't developed an alcohol-use disorder yet. In this chapter we cover what alcohol *creates or activates* in your life, the negative effects of alcohol use on your mind, body, and behavior. We explain the consequences of crossing the line repeatedly and speeding toward alcohol misuse and abuse.

People who drink in excess frequently experience psychological and cognitive difficulties. Drinking can trigger issues that were previously dormant or heighten existing problems, such as mental health disorders. New problems can also appear, like troubles with memory and judgment. Some of these issues resolve once we control our drinking, either by drinking in moderation or taking a break.

Interpersonal and relational problems are another consequence of crossing the line. It's almost impossible to maintain harmonious and rewarding bonds when you drink in excess consistently. In a relationship with a partner or spouse, drinking can take up a central negative place, deteriorating the structure of the bond. In parent-child relationships, drinking has effects on the present and the future. Work-related relationships can also be affected severely, impacting quality of life.

Health problems can be frequent when you consistently overdrink, including the struggle to maintain healthy weight and skin. We explain the reasons why we gain weight and why it's so difficult to lose even a few pounds while drinking alcohol. Although weight is only one part of the picture when it comes to overall health, it's often an important issue for women, because there are many intense social pressures related to appearance. Alcohol-related health issues can cause or intensify psychological and physical challenges in all aspects of life.

Psychological and Cognitive Effects of Alcohol

You don't need to be an alcoholic to experience the typical psychological and cognitive effects of alcohol described here. It's impossible to live your best life when you're impaired by the influence of alcohol. The good news is that most of these effects are reversible shortly after reducing or taking a break from drinking.

Alcohol Myopia

Alcohol Myopia is a concept introduced by Steele and colleagues[21] that refers to the fact that drinking alcohol decreases the amount of

---
21. Claude M. Steele and Robert A. Josephs, "Alcohol Myopia: Its Prized and Dangerous Effects." *American Psychologist*, 45 (1990): 921–933.

information a person can elaborate on. The more alcohol someone drinks, the more limited they are in the quality and quantity of the material they can pay attention to. Without alcohol, a person may be able to register the full picture of a situation, but under the influence of alcohol, they can grasp only pieces, distorted elements, or one-sided information. This can lead to an impairment in judgment.

Alcohol Myopia can affect mood as well. This is critical for women to consider, since it's been established in several studies that women's drinking is associated mainly with negative mood states. The negative mood can be connected to internal factors (e.g., feeling inadequate) or external factors (e.g., making a mistake at work), depending on which are more prominent for the person at that moment.

Difficulty Concentrating

People who drink tend to lose the focus necessary to understand a complete situation. As a result, they can experience confusion and disorganized thoughts and emotions, which can lead to distractions, delays, and poor decision-making.

Memory Problems

Alcohol affects short-term memory and especially long-term memory because it disturbs the mechanism that converts short-term into long-term memory. Gaps in memory impact all areas of functioning and can lead to delayed awareness and mistakes that affect performance.

How many times have you woken up in the morning not fully clear about what happened the night before? Even if you didn't black out, maybe you don't remember clearly what you said, who you were with, or what you posted on social media. Maybe you even see pictures on your phone that you have no recollection of taking!

Impaired Judgment

It's clear that alcohol can seriously compromise how we read situations and cause us to misstep or form wrong conclusions. This can lead to lapses of judgment in our words, actions, and decisions.

Reduced Inhibition

Since alcohol affects mood and acts on our emotions, it influences how we make sense of ourselves and interpret situations, which in turn affects how we think, act, and react. During the first or second drink, a person may feel fun, relaxed, and outgoing. But as the drinking continues, they may be all over the place, becoming more excited, aggressive, sad, or unable to think straight or maintain their boundaries.

Alcohol lowers inhibitions, and people may find themselves in circumstances or making decisions that they wouldn't consider if not under the influence of alcohol. Between this and alcohol's cognitive impacts, a woman's decision-making and behavior may be altered to such an extent that she risks finding herself in situations that are dangerous or harmful or that she regrets the next day.

Aggression

There's a known relationship between alcohol and aggression, but the specific mechanisms that underlie this relationship are not yet precisely understood. It may be connected to reduced inhibitions resulting from limited frontal lobe functioning, and to the alcohol myopia theory, which says that drinking alcohol narrows attention to the most prominent stimuli (such as angry words), with less noticeable cues being ignored.

In conclusion: Alcohol-related impairments and deficits interact, creating thoughts, behaviors, and actions that may be harmful to us and our environment. These negative outcomes may, in turn, cause us to drink more.

Relationships and Alcohol

One of the more devastating effects of alcohol misuse is how it impacts relationships, whether personal, intimate, familial, social, and work-related. It's usually the relationships closest to us that suffer the most.

The effects of alcohol are intergenerational and can be connected to relationships in the present, relationships with the generation before us (e.g., with parents, grandparents), and relationships that will continue in the near and far future (e.g., with children). The entire family system is affected. Gradually, but inevitably, alcohol consumption reduces the possibility of maintaining healthy interactions and the benefits those relationships can bring for each person involved.

Romantic and Committed Relationships

Alcohol consumption can significantly alter our personality, opening new drives and secret zones. As we start making drinking a priority, other motivations, habits, and interests gradually take second place or disappear completely. Alcohol takes center stage of everything we do, and other needs or conflicts are avoided.

Maybe you begin to hide some facts from your partner, like when and how much you drink. This can start as a subconscious or innocent defense mechanism against shame or guilt, but the secrecy might become deliberate with time. Lying, being in denial, and keeping secrets can become a way of life, part of your daily routine. Usually, the more time that passes, the more people have to lie or hide to keep things "normal." As a result, we become a different person, sometimes to the point of becoming unrecognizable to our partner and/or to ourselves, leading to tension and conflict.

As these factors continue, the partner's mistrust also grows; a *lack of confidence begins to set into the relationship.* This is the starting point where differences begin to fester. Once trust within the relationship is damaged, it's almost impossible to recover. *Open and authentic communication becomes unfeasible, which alters the foundation and possibilities of the relationship.*

Couples in this scenario are usually unhappy. Essential trust is destroyed. Arguments and fights arise about drinking or the consequences of drinking—for instance, lying, not taking responsibility for the house or the children, affairs, financial problems, neglecting crucial duties, compulsive shopping, legal problems, and so on. These conflicts trigger stress and increase the risk for mental health problems, aggression, and possibly violence and abuse.

Of course, this affects not only the couple involved but also those who live with them, such as children and parents, and other people in their family or social circle. These personal and relational problems are likely to extend into the future as well. Dysfunctional relations and communications become what's modeled for impressionable others, creating patterns and impacting future behaviors and relationships. Children who grow up in a household with significant alcohol misuse are at greater risk for developing substance use disorders themselves.

Family Relationships

When someone in a family is misusing or abusing alcohol, it affects everyone in the family. However, the reality of what's going on is usually not acknowledged or talked about. *Denial is a crucial component of an alcoholic family system.* The "family secret" has profound consequences for everyone involved, which can include:

- Worry about the health of the person who drinks.
- Fear of negative interactions, verbal abuse, conflict, or violence during or after drinking episodes.
- Feeling responsible for what's occurring.
- Feelings of guilt and/or shame.
- Confusion. There's a desire to understand what's happening or to discuss the situation, but spoken or unspoken rules determine that the family secret can't be talked about for fear of negative reprisals.
- Keeping secrets and lying to hide the family dysfunction at home, increasing tension and stress.

Impacts on Children

Parental alcohol problems impact their children in many ways. Children may clam up, become isolated, and avoid talking with others about themselves or their home life to not risk sharing anything related to their parent's drinking. They don't invite friends over to avoid unpredictable, bad situations at home or feelings of shame about their parent's drinking.

Children often misconstrue a parent's drinking as being connected to their (the child's) behavior, needs, or words (or lack thereof) and may believe that they created the problem that makes the parent drink. For some children, this leads to feelings of guilt, incapability, avoidance, and learned helplessness. Children may develop a misguided sense of obligation and accountability to care for the parent's sickness, even feeling that they're responsible to remedy it. Since they can't, they're likely to develop complicated reactions that will impact their lives in the present and future.

Children may become *angry and depressed or withdrawn* because of the suffering and neglect they experience. There's a lack of safety at home, whether emotional or physical; they may feel abandoned and not understood. They don't fully comprehend what's happening either. Heavy alcohol use disrupts some of the critical systems and situations that children depend on their parents for, to create a consistent, healthy, nurturing environment. For example:

- *Parents' psychological state and behaviors.* Under the influence of alcohol, parents may change their behavior, mood or language. Children are unlikely to understand or know how to make sense of this; many children think the change in adult behavior is their fault, that they did or said something that provoked these mood swings.
- *Consistent daily routines,* such as mealtimes, hygiene, bedtimes, evening and weekend activities, homework, preparation for school, family rituals—all of which are crucial for healthy growth and mental health.

Without consistency and predictability, it's challenging for a kid to experience safe boundaries and to grow in a healthy way. We all need a stable platform from which to develop. Without it, the natural reaction is to pay attention to the *cracks in the current situation* instead of looking to progress and succeed in the future. Unfortunately, the primary response of children in these situations of neglect, abandonment, lack of health, and attachment/relationship modeling is some combination of shame, guilt, frustration, helplessness, and anger.

Early ways of relating to our primary caregivers can influence how we connect later in life with partners, friends, coworkers, family members, and especially children. Negative feelings that started with a drinking parent may pop up to create difficulties in these future relationships.

At this point you may think, *"My situation is not this bad. I'm still engaged with my children and have my home life under control."* Indeed, it's possible that this is your situation currently. However, we can make four observations here:

1. It's difficult to overestimate how extremely sensitive children can be, especially regarding feelings they may link with a problem they don't understand, which in their minds also makes it an area of unpredictability and therefore more dangerous.

2. Situations can quickly become associated with a parent drinking, even if this isn't the case. Say, a parent is sick with the flu and unable to take the child to school. The child may make sense of this by remembering another instance of "being sick" connected to *the problem that has no name* (crossing the line with alcohol), and associate the current event with alcohol, even if they're unrelated.

3. Children remember things they don't understand for a long time, sometimes forever. Situations and episodes related to the parent's drinking may remain in the child's mind and might affect them in a conscious, subconscious, or unconscious way for the rest of their life.

4. Children of parents that cross the line at home have the tendency to start drinking during the teenage years and often have several binge drinking episodes at an early age.[22,23,24] When parents drink heavily, some of the consequences their children suffer include hyperactivity and emotional problems in childhood, psychological and behavioral problems in adolescence, and alcoholism in adulthood.[25]

---

22. Louise Hayes et al., "Parenting Influences on Adolescent Use," *Australian Institute of Family Studies* (2004): 70.
23. Conor Gilligan and Kypros Kypri, "Parent Attitudes, Family Dynamics and Adolescent Drinking: Qualitative Study of the Australian Parenting Guidelines for Adolescent Alcohol Use," *BMC Public Health* 12 (2012): 7.
24. "Parents May Be Putting Their Children on a Path to Drinking," *National Drug and Alcohol Research Centre (NDARC)*, published September 8, 2014, accessed August 2023, https://ndarc.med.unsw.edu.au/news/parents-may-be-putting-their-children-path-drinking.
25. Hayes et al., "Parenting Influences on Adolescent Use"; Gilligan and Kypri, "Parent Attitudes, Family Dynamics and Adolescent Drinking"; NDARC, published September 8, 2014.

Even if the situation created by your drinking *"isn't that bad,"* we guarantee that problems will arise that carry over into your relationship with your kids in the short or long term. Drinking often and in excess becomes more frequent, with worse effects every time, for the simple reason that *alcohol is addictive.* You can develop more tolerance to it than others, but alcohol dependence will affect and limit you in the long run. *Your children are aware of your drinking, even if you act normal and everything looks okay.* They perceive the smell of alcohol in your breath, they know about your drinking routines, and they're concerned about your emotional dependence on alcohol even if not at the level of clear conscious awareness.

Think about it...
1. Do you drink when your kids are present?
2. Have you had a conversation with your children regarding your drinking? How did it go? Are they aware of how much you drink?
3. Have you had any conversation or confrontation with your kids while under the influence of alcohol that you would like to take back?
4. Have you experienced a situation you regret? What can you do to prevent another situation like that?

Work Relationships

Two main types of problems bubble up at the intersection of work life and crossing the line with alcohol.

The first is *underperformance* due to hangovers, absenteeism, and presenteeism. Presenteeism refers to the low productivity that happens when employees aren't fully present and effective at work. Alcohol affects current and potential performance since it has a ripple effect on developing capabilities and expertise.

The second is a *propensity to make mistakes*. Employees who drink are more likely to make errors and not perform their duties fully. Making unnecessary mistakes affects self-confidence and damages trust and relationships with supervisors and colleagues. As a result, the person is less likely to progress in their career, which can impact their earning potential and subsequent quality of life.

Think about it …
1. How many times in the last six months have you taken a sick day at work due to drinking?
2. How many days per week and per month are you hungover?
3. Have you noticed making more mistakes or feeling awkward in your interactions with colleagues because you drank in excess the night before?

Financial Troubles

Due to lowered inhibitions and poor judgment that stem from crossing the line with alcohol, we become prone to making unnecessary purchases. Or we spend hours at bars or restaurants, where drinks are three times more expensive than at home. Credit card statements may come with a lot of unexplained charges.

> *"I drink almost every day, but I take it easy, no more than two glasses of wine. However, on Fridays, after a long week, I enjoy going to a restaurant with friends. Usually, I spend around $20.00 on the food, and not less than $45.00 on drinks. With the tip, it runs to almost $80.00 for a mediocre dinner!"* —Tamara

On another level, there are remarkably high costs for alcohol-related consequences like a DWI. If there are accidents under the influence, a person will find themselves in big trouble, especially if others are affected or injured, or if there's property damage. Resolving a DWI with an attorney's assistance can be costly, and there are serious future consequences related to a DWI, even when there's no injury or damage. On top of that, there's an economic responsibility not only for the person who caused the accident but also potentially for their spouse since the law sees spouses as a financial unit.

The Problem of Losing Weight

"The difficult story with my weight started when I was in my late twenties. At that time I was married and had an excellent job. We didn't want children yet, so my social life was pretty intense. Alcohol was everywhere—parties, restaurants, birthdays, holidays, even baby showers. I became a little overweight, not bad, but enough to feel disappointed with myself.

"The major problem was dressing up every day. I felt that nothing looked good on me, especially skirts, shorts, or swimsuits. I felt ashamed. My self-esteem hit the floor, and I lost joy and excitement, even though my life was good. I tried different diets, I started working out, but nothing happened. I didn't drop a pound. Actually, very gradually, my weight was going up.

"I started feeling a disconnection with my husband, that his interest in spending time with me was going down. I found out he was having an affair. I was so sad and felt betrayed. I started drinking more to cope with the situation. And, of course, the problem with my weight got worse." —Adrienne

Chapter 3: What Happens When You Cross the Line

There are several reasons why drinking makes it difficult to lose weight and could lead to gradually gaining more weight.

1. *Alcohol contains "empty" calories:* Alcohol contains calories, but the calories in alcohol don't have nutritional value or nourishing substances (hence the "empty" calories). On top of that, calories from alcohol are burned first, before your body uses calories from anything else. This means that the lipids from fats and the glucose from carbohydrates of other foods you've eaten don't get used up; they become "excess," which then becomes fatty tissue.

2. *Alcohol adds calories to your diet:* There are a lot of calories in alcoholic drinks. A standard wine pour is 5 ounces (150 ml), which contains about 120 calories; the average serving of beer is 12 ounces (350 ml) with 150 calories. A night out can mean adding hundreds, if not thousands, of extra calories to your body, on top of the calories from food. Think about how many glasses of wine you can drink on a night out—three, four or more? You may be adding over 400 extra calories depending on what and how much you drink on each occasion.

3. *Alcohol leads to poor food choices:* During and after drinking, especially late at night or during a hangover, people are more inclined to eat foods or snacks that are higher in fats or sugars, without really noticing it (impaired judgment is happening here, too). Some research suggests that alcohol leads to an increase in food intake, making us eat more food and more frequently.[26] Your drinking may be sabotaging your intentions to maintain a healthy diet and weight.

4. *Alcohol slows metabolism:* The body can't store alcohol and must metabolize it immediately, so the metabolism[27] of sugars and fats from

---
26. Martin R. Yeomans, Samantha Caton, and Marion M. Hetherington, "Alcohol and Food Intake," *Current Opinion in Clinical Nutrition and Metabolic Care* 6, no. 6 (November 2023): 639–644, doi: 10.1097/00075197-200311000-00006. PMID: 14557794.
27. Metabolism is the body's process of absorbing, breaking down, and eliminating substances in the body.

food you eat takes second place. Your body will redirect the energy that breaks down carbs and fats and burns those calories and use it instead to process the alcohol you ingested.

5. *Alcohol slows your physical activity:* When you start drinking, your energy and vitality take a dip, which continues for several hours, sometimes until the following day. As a result, you may not be burning calories to either lose weight or maintain your healthy weight.

In the next section, Dr. William Triplett speaks from his extensive experience on how drinking alcohol is damaging our health, opening our eyes to the destructive power alcohol has on women's lives, and building awareness on how to have a healthy life that reverses the damage alcohol causes.

How Alcohol Damages Our Health and How to Reverse the Damage
By Dr. Triplett

To feel well and thrive as a human being, several conditions must be in place. These are the lifestyle determinants of health:[28] proper nutrition, adequate sleep, regular physical exercise, avoiding harmful substances, managing stress, and maintaining healthy relationships.

Alcohol can have harmful effects on each of these lifestyle determinants of health, and each of these determinants affects the others. For example, alcohol intake results in poor-quality sleep. Over time, this can become sleep deprivation, which can lead to fatigue, irregular eating,

---

28. "6 Ways to Take Control of Your Health: Lifestyle Medicine," *American College of Lifestyle Medicine*, 2023, accessed May 5, 2023, https://lifestylemedicine.org/wp-content/uploads/2023/06/Pillar-Booklet.pdf.

overeating, and weight gain. Weight gain and poor sleep can lead to, or increase, feelings of depression and anxiety. Depression causes withdrawal from social contact and decreased motivation, including to exercise. Decreased exercise and social isolation lead to decreased stress tolerance. All these factors increase the chance that we will use and abuse substances such as alcohol, tobacco, and other drugs. So it goes in a complicated web of causes and effects that leads to a downward spiral in our health and ability to be happy.

Our habits have a huge effect on these determinants. This is great news, because it means that we have the chance to choose and act differently, to change our habits. Most women don't see the effects that alcohol is having on their well-being. It's not until they give alcohol up for a month, two months, or even longer that they see how good they can feel. As the toxins from alcohol leave their bodies, their cells, tissues, and organs heal, and their function returns to normal.

All of us want to feel well. We want to be free from pain, sadness, and suffering. We want to be vibrant, happy, and full of energy. We want to enjoy life to the fullest. In my career as a family physician, I have spent most of the past twenty-plus years trying to help my patients feel their best and improve their function. Unfortunately, our habits and lifestyles play a big part in creating our suffering.

In this part of the chapter, we'll look more closely at the effects of alcohol on the brain and body from a medical perspective. I'll discuss a bit of the history of alcohol use, how the scientific opinion about the safety of alcohol use is changing, and the effects of alcohol on the human body and brain. I'll introduce the topic of Alcohol Use Disorder. We close the chapter with four case studies.

Human beings discovered drinking alcohol or ethanol more than 9,000 years ago. Every culture with written history has documented the effects of its use, including the downsides. This work continues today, with recent headlines announcing the discovery that drinking the equivalent of one-half beer per day leads to a measurable decrease in the size of the human brain.[29] In January 2022, the World Heart Federation (WHF) released a new policy brief that questioned the idea that moderate alcohol consumption is healthy for the cardiovascular system.[30] The WHF pointed to the flawed design of the original studies from decades ago that were touted by the alcohol industry and individuals who daily use alcohol. For several decades, media outlets have also claimed that moderate alcohol drinking has health benefits, particularly in reducing cardiovascular events such as heart attacks and strokes. Now, this information is being questioned and even refuted by scientists and physicians.

The WHF advises that no alcohol should be considered safe for human consumption, and that any amount of alcohol diminishes an individual's health. They support this claim with statistics on the harmful effects of alcohol. In 2019, 2.4 million people died worldwide because of alcohol-related problems, accounting for 4.3 percent of all deaths. Alcohol has long been a significant contributor to avoidable diseases and injuries, including cardiovascular disease, cancer, gastrointestinal illness, accidental injuries, and violence-related deaths.

For all recorded history, men have used and abused more alcohol than women. But over the past one hundred years, women in the US have been closing the gap on drinking prevalence, total alcohol consumed, frequency of binge drinking, diagnosis of Alcohol Use

---
29. Remi Daviet et al., "Associations between Alcohol Consumption and Gray and White Matter Volumes in the UK Biobank," *Nature Communications* 13, no. 1 (March 4, 2022): 1–11, https://doi.org/10.1038/s41467-022-28735-5.
30. "The Impact of Alcohol on Cardiovascular Health: Myths and Measures," *World Heart Federation*, published January 20, 2022, accessed May 2023, https://world-heart-federation.org/news/no-amount-of-alcohol-is-good-for-the-heart-says-world-heart-federation/.

Disorder, and early-onset drinking.[31] This trend has accelerated over the past ten years.

For women, alcohol-related deaths doubled between 1999 and 2017. Alcohol contributed to 15–20 percent of drug overdoses, 26 percent of suicides, and 50 percent of liver-related deaths. The increase in alcohol-associated deaths was greater in women than in men. The greatest increase occurred in women ages 25–34. Alcohol use increased in every age group for women. Young women (age 25–29) and older women (age greater than 60) increased their alcohol consumption more than males of the same ages.[32]

At equal doses of alcohol, women suffer more negative effects than men. They're at greater risk for experiencing the toxic effects of alcohol, because they have lower average body weight, reduced body water, and slower alcohol metabolism as compared to men. They experience more hangovers, blackouts, liver damage, brain atrophy, cognitive deficits, heart damage, injuries, and death. Women also progress faster in developing alcohol use disorder and are less likely to seek treatment for alcohol addiction than men. Increased drinking during the COVID-19 pandemic caused many women and men to progress from occasional or heavy drinking to Alcohol Use Disorder. Drinking alcohol to cope with stress and anxiety and relieve emotional pain places many women on the fast track to alcohol addiction. Overall, the poisonous impacts of alcohol are higher for women.

The definition of a standard drink is 12 ounces of regular beer (5% alcohol), 5 ounces of wine (10–15% alcohol), or 1.5 ounces of spirits (40% alcohol). Heavy drinking for women means drinking eight or more standard drinks in a week (fifteen is the cutoff for men).

---

31. George F. Koob, "Keynote: 'Alcohol and the Female Brain,'" *2017 National Conference on Alcohol and Opioid Use in Women and Girls: Advances in Prevention, Treatment and Recovery Research*, presented October 27, 2017.
32. Aaron M. White, I-Jen P. Castle, Ralph W. Hingson, and Patricia A. Powell, "Using Death Certificates to Explore Changes in Alcohol-Related Mortality in the United States, 1999 to 2017," Alcoholism: Clinical and Experimental Research 44, no. 1 (January 7, 2020): 178-187, https://doi.org/10.1111/acer.14239.

Many drinkers underestimate how much alcohol they have imbibed. Few people measure their hard alcohol, and restaurants and bars frequently serve portions twice the standard drink size. Beers and wines vary in their alcohol compositions, and bartenders pour them in containers with different volumes.

The Centers for Disease Control and Prevention (CDC) keep detailed statistics on the harmful effects of alcohol. The Alcohol-Related Death Index lists the diseases, injuries, and deaths wholly caused by, or related to, alcohol consumption.[33] These are listed below and detailed on the CDC website.

- Alcohol abuse
- Alcohol dependence
- Alcoholic cardiomyopathy
- Alcoholic gastritis
- Alcoholic polyneuropathy
- Alcoholic liver disease
- Alcoholic myopathy
- Alcoholic psychosis
- Pancreatitis, acute and chronic
- Esophageal varices
- Gallbladder disease
- Gastrointestinal hemorrhage
- Liver cirrhosis
- Hepatitis
- Infant death
- Premature birth
- Small for gestational age birth
- Low birth weight
- Neonatal pneumonia

---

33. "Effects of Drinking Alcohol on Your Health," *CDC: Alcohol Portal*, page last reviewed September 14, 2022, accessed May 5, 2023, https://www.cdc.gov/alcoholportal/.

- Neonatal seizures
- Breast cancer
- Colorectal cancer
- Esophageal cancer
- Laryngeal cancer
- Liver cancer
- Oropharyngeal cancer
- Pancreatic cancer
- Prostate cancer
- Stomach cancer
- Atrial fibrillation
- Coronary artery disease
- Hypertension
- Stroke
- Alcohol poisoning
- Motor vehicle crash
- Suicide
- Child maltreatment
- Drowning
- Falls
- Fire
- Firearm accidents
- Homicide
- Work injuries
- Hypothermia

About 90 percent of people who drink alcohol don't meet the criteria for an alcohol use disorder. Alcohol use disorders separate into mild, moderate, and severe categories. The gold standard for diagnosing an alcohol use disorder is the criteria contained in the Diagnostic and Statistical Manual of Mental Disorders (DSM-5-TR).[34] People with severe alcohol use disorder would formerly be referred to as alcoholics or having alcohol dependence. Some signs of severe alcohol use disorder (AUD) include:

- Inability to limit drinking.
- Continuing to drink despite personal or professional problems.
- Needing to drink more and more to get the same effect.
- Wanting a drink so badly that you can't think of anything else.

Addiction can be defined as the continual and compulsive consumption of a substance or behavior despite its harm to self and/or others. Many people recognize that their drinking is a problem before they meet the criteria for AUD, before they become addicted. They recognize the harm alcohol is causing to their physical and mental health, relationships, and performance. These people can frequently give up alcohol entirely by changing their mind about alcohol and then changing their behavior.

How does alcohol affect the human body and brain? Alcohol has widespread effects on the body and particularly on the brain.[35] These effects are seen even at low doses of alcohol. When we consume alcohol, it's rapidly absorbed in the gastrointestinal tract, especially the small intestine. The stomach absorbs some alcohol, and even the mouth and esophagus absorb small amounts. Absorption is accelerated by carbonation (such as beer) and an empty stomach. The alcohol then enters the bloodstream, where a large portion passes through the liver.

In the body, alcohol is metabolized to acetaldehyde primarily by the liver but also in other tissues. This acetaldehyde damages the cells

---

34. *American Psychiatric Association* (2013).
35. Joseph Loscalzo et al., *Harrison's Principles of Internal Medicine*, 21st ed. (McGraw Hill, 2022).

and tissues by increasing inflammation and free radicals inside the cell. Acetaldehyde poisons the cells, and they must do all they can to eliminate it quickly. The cells' enzymes are hijacked for a time to do this work and must abandon their normal functions. A small amount of alcohol, from 2–10 percent of what's consumed, is excreted in the breath, sweat, and urine without being processed.

When ethanol enters the bloodstream, it takes only five minutes to reach your brain's tissues, where it has its most profound effects. Alcohol is primarily a depressant drug causing decreased neuron activity. This effect is similar to that of benzodiazepines, barbiturates, and other sedatives.

Alcohol enters the brain and stimulates the pleasure centers to release dopamine. This dopamine release is the same release that occurs with many different chemical and natural stimuli. Dopamine release is related to motivational control and seeking states to gain a reward; for example, it happens when you're hungry and find food, when you're thirsty and find water, or when you're cold and find warm shelter. This same response also occurs with most intoxicating drugs, including cocaine, methamphetamine, and heroin. The reaction of dopamine release with alcohol and other drugs is much stronger than with nondrug rewards.

Different people get different degrees of reward response to alcohol use, which may account for an individual's motivation to take another drink. Genetics and other factors determine the variety of reactions in the brain to a dose of alcohol. One person gets a significant dopamine response with their first drink of alcohol and finds it extremely pleasant. They also notice a numbing of negative emotional states. This person wants to drink alcohol again. They ignore the adverse effects of intoxication. The road to addiction to alcohol starts here. A second person experiences only a tiny dopamine response. They instead notice more of the painful effects of the alcohol, like a hangover, and will be less likely to want more. This person goes out with friends for dinner, orders one beer, and drinks only half. They're less likely to experience future alcohol-related problems.

The person prone to alcohol addiction desires to drink again soon. The initial dose of alcohol caused them to feel great by either giving them a high or taking away their pain for a while. They try it again, and the same response happens. The episodes repeatedly occur while a subtle change occurs in the brain: The same dose of alcohol gives less joy and less relief from pain as time passes. We fix this "problem" by increasing the dose. But the target state we seek continues to move. We drink more and more, and the toxic effects of alcohol begin to be a problem. Alcohol-related problems tend to be progressive in nature: binge drinking, hangovers, blackouts, and withdrawal symptoms.

The Binge and Hangover

Meagan took a swig from a beer bottle and made a face. She stood in her bathroom dressed in her underwear. She frowned as she applied mascara carefully. The frown arose with the thought that she looked ugly and fat. Her eyes were red and looked puffy. She practiced a flirty smile in the mirror, and then her face relaxed back to a frown. Her belly stuck out more than she liked.

She had always struggled to keep her weight down. She dragged herself to spin class, hot yoga, and boot camp after work so that she could let loose on the weekend and party with her friends. She sighed and made a mental note to work out harder next week and double down on her diet. No sugar! She knew that alcohol had a lot of calories and could cause weight gain, so she was careful with her diet and exercise routine during the week—the picture of healthy living. Since she was young, her mother had emphasized staying thin. She had encouraged her to "drink like a lady," whatever that meant.

Chapter 3: What Happens When You Cross the Line

Meagan slipped into her short sleeveless dress and sucked in her stomach. *Good enough*, she thought, and put on her shoes. Her head throbbed, and she felt dizzy when she bent over. She sat still for a minute and finished her beer.

Preparing for Saturday night challenged her every week because it repeated Friday night. She and her friends pre-gamed before going clubbing. They'd drink a couple of shots at one of their houses, then go out to dance and drink some more until the early morning hours. This was Friday and Saturday night every week, going back at least since she'd left college five years ago. As an independent working woman, Meagan loved the freedom of being young and single and having a bright future. She worked hard every week and played hard on the weekends.

But she noticed that she felt terrible on Saturdays and Sundays. She laughed about this with her friends, trading hangover stories and remedies. She believed only in her dad's treatment, "the hair of the dog,"[36] thus the beer sipping while getting ready to go out. To recover, Meagan slept till noon on the weekend, rolled out of bed, took four ibuprofen, and washed it down with a beer. An hour later, she felt almost human. She hated the taste of beer, but thought it was necessary. She and her girlfriends stuck to "skinny drinks" at the clubs, such as vodka with a splash of cranberry.

Meagan and her girlfriends all had similar stories. Their lives resembled reality TV shows with all the drama and angst. Their weekend misadventures included falling down the stairs at the club, vomiting in the bathroom, and lying on the floor crying for hours. They laughed about near misses while driving, blackouts, and hookups with cute and not so cute guys. The drama between the friends existed as a constant theme. There was always someone angry with someone else, always some undercurrent of jealousy and resentment.

---

36. As per Merriam-Webster, the idiom the "hair of the dog (that bit you)" refers to "an alcoholic drink that is taken by someone to feel better after having drunk too much at an earlier time."

Meagan would reflect on this sometimes and consider backing off, settling down a bit. She didn't enjoy this spectacle anymore; she didn't feel happy or high when she was drunk. But she knew that for a while each Friday and Saturday night, her anxiety was totally gone. She felt the pressures of life disappear with her third or fourth drink. On to five, six, or seven and then complete numbness. She never kept count anymore. If she was asked, she'd always give a number she judged to be not too high to worry her friends and not too low to lose their respect.

You can probably tell that Meagan and her friends are binge drinkers. Binge drinking is one example of excessive alcohol use.[37] When women drink four or more drinks on a single occasion, we call it a binge, mainly if the drinking is done in two hours or less and the blood alcohol content (BAC) rises above 0.08 percent, the level used to delineate DUI (driving under the influence). In men, the cutoff for a binge is five drinks. Binge drinking leads to intoxication or drunkenness. Another category, High-Intensity Drinking, means drinking eight drinks on one occasion for women and ten for men. This type of drinking is prevalent among young adults, especially those attending college.

Meagan and her friends are at a higher risk of developing alcohol use disorder and complications from intoxication and alcohol poisoning. Around 22 percent of women Meagan's age report an episode of binge drinking in the past month.[38] Binge drinking among women is on the rise. In the US, more than 140,000 people die from excess alcohol intake per year, and 46 percent of these deaths were associated with binge drinking.[39]

---

37. CDC uses the term "excessive alcohol use" to include binge drinking, heavy drinking, underage drinking, and alcohol use during pregnancy.
38. "Alcohol Effects on Health: Research-Based Information on Drinking and Its Impact," *NIAAA*, accessed May 5, 2023, https://www.niaaa.nih.gov/alcohols-effects-health.
39. "Deaths from Excessive Alcohol Use in the United States," *CDC*, last reviewed July 6, 2022, accessed May 5, 2023, https://www.cdc.gov/alcohol/features/excessive-alcohol-deaths.html.

Binge drinking has many other harmful effects, including slowed reaction time, decreased coordination, poor balance, poor judgment, and slurred speech. These effects are responsible for increasing injuries and deaths with alcohol, including motor vehicle crashes, falls, violence-related injuries, and suicide. Alcohol poisons all human tissue, and repeated binge drinking can lead to many chronic diseases, including neurologic disorders, gastrointestinal diseases, and many types of cancer. Binge drinking can lead to alcohol poisoning, coma, and death.

Heavy drinking and binge drinking can lead to weight gain and difficulty losing weight. This relationship between alcohol and weight is complex and involves many factors, including genetics, physical activity level, sleeping habits, and behavioral traits. Of course, not all heavy drinkers are overweight, and not all overweight people are heavy drinkers.

There are several reasons for why heavy drinking leads to weight gain for many women. Alcohol impairs judgment, and this leads to overeating and poor food choices during or after drinking. People who are prone to binge drinking are frequently prone to binge eating as well.

Alcohol has seven calories per gram and no nutritional value. Heavy drinkers get a high percentage of their daily calories from alcohol, but these are "empty calories," because they don't provide anything useful that the body needs, like minerals, vitamins, fats, or protein.. Many beers contain a lot of carbohydrates, and liquors are commonly mixed with sugary sodas or juices. Heavy beer consumption can lead to increased abdominal fat (sometimes called beer belly), especially in men.

Alcohol use leads to poor sleep, which contributes to weight gain in adults. Both poor sleep and alcohol use increase depression symptoms. Depression can lead to unhealthy eating patterns. Alcohol also hijacks the drinker's metabolism, stopping the liver from burning fats for energy. The liver must process all the alcohol to remove the toxins from the body before it returns to normal functions.

Meagan suffers from hangovers after each episode of binge drinking. Being hungover the next day is common for pretty much anyone who binge drinks. Hangover symptoms usually last for several hours and include headaches, intense thirst, increased blood pressure, anxiety, sensitivity to sound and light, body aches, and dizziness. Alcohol causes hangovers by various mechanisms, including dehydration, disrupted sleep, irritation of the gastrointestinal tract, and inflammation in body tissues caused by acetaldehyde.

There's also the possibility of having a case of mini-withdrawal after each episode of bingeing, which is similar to what heavy daily drinkers experience each time their blood alcohol level goes down. They lose the calm feeling they get when their alcohol level increases. Anxiety and restlessness replace positive emotions. Hangover symptoms last about twenty-four hours, and there's no cure for them other than to hydrate, sleep, eat nutritious food, and wait for the body to clear all the toxins.

The Spiral

Cate arrives home after another stressful day at work. She sets her purse on the kitchen table and yells a quick hello to her children. "Hi, mom," they shout from another room. She walks straight to the fridge and takes out a chilled bottle of chardonnay. This moment has been on her mind since she got to work this morning. She gives herself a generous pour and takes the first sip, then a second. Only now does she hang up her coat, put on her best smile, and greet her children in person.

While the kids talk about their day at school, Cate struggles with the urge to return to her glass in the kitchen. The stress of her day is still with her, her brain cycling between the pressures of work, marriage, parenting, housework: she has the complete "adulting" package. She knows that soon, she'll be able to let all this go for a short while. The pain and pressure will evaporate somewhere into her second bottle of wine, about the time she finishes cooking dinner and her husband gets home. Her brain will be turned off, the stress melted, the mind numbed. But she knows that these feelings will return when she wakes up tomorrow. She wonders how she got to this place in her life.

Her life has repeated in the same way each day for several years now. She wakes up every morning feeling like crap. Her head hurts. Everything hurts. She feels tired and weak, sad and nervous simultaneously. She doesn't remember ever feeling good. She drags herself from bed, makes coffee, and gets in the shower. She prepares for work and gets the kids ready for school. The numbness from last night is completely gone, and she feels anxious about the day ahead, work meetings, her kids, her marriage, and all the many responsibilities and pressures that come with trying to make life function. It takes all of her will and fortitude to survive each day. She walks to her car in the garage and notices the recycling box overflowing with wine bottles. She feels a brief pang of guilt but starts counting down the hours until she can turn off her brain again and escape.

Cate demonstrates all the stages of addiction described by Koob and Volkow.[40] Alcohol may no longer give her euphoria or a high now that she has been drinking heavily for years. Her brain wiring has changed with repeated exposure to alcohol. Her baseline mood has been reset to a constant negative mental state that's very close to depression accompanied by anxiety. She feels no pleasure in life from the normal joys of the human experience. Vacations, date nights with her husband, the beauty of nature, and the joy of art and music give her no happiness. The

---
40. George F. Koob and Nora D. Volkow, "Neurobiology of Addiction: A Neurocircuitry Analysis," *The Lancet Psychiatry* 3, no. 8 (August 2016): 760–773.

only thing that gives her any temporary relief is alcohol. The amount of alcohol it takes to experience that relief has increased with time.

What has happened to Cate, without her realization, is that she's now entering a state of alcohol withdrawal every day, making her feel physically ill and emotionally distraught. She thinks about drinking earlier and earlier in the day. She plans her evenings carefully and makes sure she has two bottles of wine each night. At times she recognizes that her drinking has become a problem. She plans to cut back and make healthy changes in her life. She sees that her relationships are suffering. She has watched her career stagnate as her motivation to work has disappeared. But she's tired, her will falters, and she stays trapped in a downward spiral.

Now that we know about the hazards of alcohol use, and what it does to our bodies and brains, we should look at two possible outcomes in the story of a woman who crosses the line into a severe AUD and a second woman who chooses an alcohol-free life.

Losing It All

Sophia fumbled with her key fob as she walked to her car. Her hands were shaking violently now; she was sweating and felt dizzy and anxious. Her work break had been delayed by an hour, and she could feel it. She grabbed the bottle from under the driver's seat as she sat down to take a long drink. Cheap vodka at ten in the morning. This was her life now. She finished the first half of the bottle and took a deep breath. She was coming back to normal. Not *normal normal*—she hadn't felt normal in decades. Her version of normal was just feeling less sick, well enough to show up to work checking groceries at her local supermarket.

She reflected briefly on how different her life had become. Her marriage, her family, a good career—one by one, she had lost all of them years ago. Her alcohol use led to the end of her marriage, and her kids had gone no contact. She had been to jail for a DUI. Word of her alcohol abuse got around, and this reputation prevented her from continuing in her field as a banker.

Sophia felt disgusted with herself but powerless to make any changes. She had quit drinking alcohol on her own many times, but this was years ago. Now the only time she quit drinking was the five or six hours a night that she was asleep. She glanced at her watch; break was almost over. She took a final drink from the bottle and replaced it under her seat. She'd left enough for a few drinks for her afternoon break and worried that it wasn't enough. She would be shaking again by her next break.

Sophia's symptoms meet the criteria for a severe alcohol use disorder according to the DSM-5. (This condition used to be called alcohol dependence or alcoholism.) The criteria for AUD include:

- Recurrent drinking resulting in failure to fulfill role obligations.
- Recurrent drinking in hazardous situations.
- Continued drinking despite alcohol-related social or interpersonal problems.
- Evidence of tolerance.
- Evidence of alcohol withdrawal or use of alcohol for relief or avoidance of withdrawal.
- Drinking in larger amounts or over longer periods than intended.
- Persistent desire or unsuccessful attempts to reduce or stop drinking.
- Spending a great deal of time obtaining, using, or recovering from alcohol.
- Giving up or reducing important activities because of drinking.
- Continued drinking despite knowledge of physical or psychological problems created by alcohol.
- Alcohol craving.

Mild AUD can usually be treated with outpatient counseling and/or group therapy programs. Moderate to severe AUD may require a more structured treatment program and medications. This book and program aren't intended as a substitute for the standard treatments for those with AUD. People with AUD should seek the care of an appropriate medical professional. This book and program are directed to those with problem drinking that could lead to the development of AUD over time and to those who might be motivated to give up alcohol to maximize their physical and psychological health.

Alcohol Free

Paula's heart pounded in her chest. She struggled to catch her breath as she approached the peak. She hadn't climbed this hill for many years. A smile came to her lips despite the physical discomfort she experienced from the uphill hike.

She stopped and surveyed the scene. The clear blue sky extended in all directions from her vantage point to the horizon. She noticed the warmth of the sun on her face and a cooling breeze on her back. Her legs burned from the climb, a pain that she wouldn't have tolerated a year ago, but now registered in her mind as a satisfying use of her muscles. So many things appeared to her as pleasant now, a hundred or more small joys every day. Paula was grateful for these joys. Her mind felt as clear as the blue sky she viewed from the top of the hill. She felt so alive!

For several years the sky of her mind had been dark and cloudy, seemingly darker each year. Her mood mirrored this; she'd lost hope for the future. Paula medicated her symptoms with alcohol for many years and received less and less relief as time went on. After many failed attempts at cutting back on her drinking, it became clear to her that more drastic action was needed. She resolved to quit alcohol completely and for good.

After two weeks with no alcohol, Paula noticed many changes in her health. She slept well and woke up feeling refreshed. Her mood improved, subtly at first, but week by week, she was brighter and more open. She began to think about the future with hope and anticipation.

Her energy level improved, and she began a walking program, starting at ten minutes a day and gradually increasing to thirty minutes or more. Now she walks at least three miles a day with her dog and frequently goes on hikes of seven to ten miles on weekend days. She has started yoga classes three times a week.

Paula became interested in her health and made it a priority. She regained her interest in cooking and now pays careful attention to her diet. Her digestion improved dramatically, and the stomach pains she'd had for years resolved.

Paula has watched her relationships improve. She was interested more in other people and reached out to old friends. She cut ties with friends who were not open to, or understanding of, her changed relationship with alcohol.

When she looks in the mirror, a happier, younger-looking Paula smiles back at her. The whites of her eyes are clearer; the redness and blotchy skin transformed into a healthy glow. She feels like a new person since quitting alcohol one year ago.

Paula's story may sound like a miracle, but for decades, physicians and scientists have been aware of the ability of the liver and other internal organs to repair and regenerate after alcohol cessation. During alcohol use, the liver becomes infiltrated with fat and then chronically inflamed. Over time, this leads to scarring and loss of healthy liver tissue called fibrosis. The liver then can become cirrhotic and fail, leading to death. With alcohol abstinence, the fatty liver can return to normal, and fibrosis and cirrhosis can improve.[41] Healthy liver tissue regenerates to a degree.

This tissue healing and repair occurs in other parts of the gastrointestinal tract, too. Chronic pancreatitis improves or sometimes heals completely. Inflammation in the intestinal tract improves, and the intestinal barrier heals. The disruption in the normal microbiota of the intestines also can recover with time. This means more healthy bugs in your gut, which help with digestion and many other aspects of health, including mood and immune function. Nutrients that couldn't be absorbed by the damaged intestines during alcohol use are now taken up by the gut and help heal the body and mind.

Muscles and bones also become healthier and stronger when we quit alcohol. These improvements are multiplied when we add an exercise routine to the recovery process. The accelerated aging of the skin caused by alcohol stops with abstinence, and it's common for people to appear younger and healthier when they quit alcohol. The ability of the tissues and cells of the body to recover from chronic poisoning is quite miraculous.

We know that the brains of heavy alcohol users are smaller and less dense than those of nonalcohol users. This difference can be seen in standard brain imaging, including CT and MRI scans. Drinking one-half beer per day on average causes this measurable brain shrinkage over time. Brain volume and density increase toward normal when people quit alcohol, demonstrating the amazing healing capacity of the brain.

More recent and exciting news about brain healing with alcohol cessation comes from pictures via functional MRI and PET (tests that show brain activity by location by measuring blood flow and metab-

---

41. "Alcohol Effects on Health," *NIAAA*, accessed May 5, 2023.

olism) scans of the brain. The brains of people who don't drink and those with alcohol use disorders differ significantly in the areas of the brain responsible for executive function (the cortex) and balance and coordination (the cerebellum). There's reduced activity in these areas in the brains of alcohol users. But these abnormalities partially reverse with abstinence! Although they may not reverse completely, tests of brain function show that long-term abstinence is associated with the return of normal cognitive function in all but the most severe cases of alcohol abuse. Scientists believe that the brain is rewiring during abstinence, bypassing circuits damaged by alcohol use, so that the same functions are accomplished with different neural pathways. The slowest function to recover is the visuospatial function.[42]

Quitting alcohol sooner leads to better and more complete healing. Paula's story shows a typical recovery after becoming alcohol-free; it's not exaggerated. When we stop poisoning our brains and bodies, the healing begins, and we come back to the path that leads to our best selves.

---

42. The ability to assemble furniture with the help of a line diagram is an example of visuospatial function.

Notes:

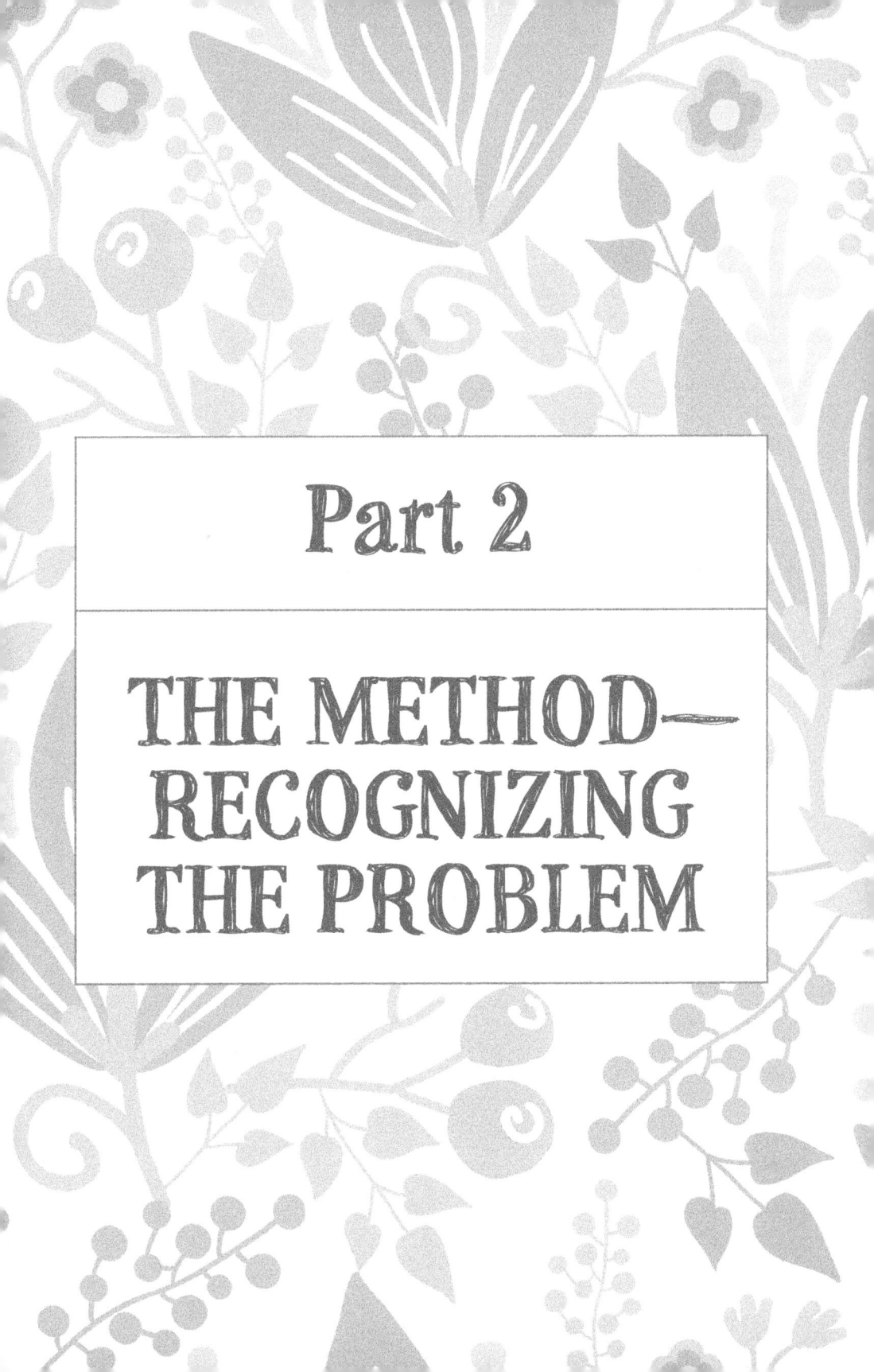

Part 2

THE METHOD— RECOGNIZING THE PROBLEM

Part 2: The Method

Our method is based on helping you to reconsider your drinking. A big part of this is enhancing your ability *to think critically and for yourself about your drinking based on your personal values and hopes for your life*, rather than falling back on what society in general tells us about drinking or going with the flow of peer pressure or popular norms.

To make an effective change, you must focus on what you're going *to gain* as a result of that change. Focusing on what you think you're going to lose or miss out on—for example, alcohol, friends, your personality when you drink, "fun" at social events, etc.—will prevent you from making a decision.

It's vital *to establish a positive mindset* toward reclaiming your freedom from the grip of drinking and societal messaging about alcohol. That way, you'll be able to regain control and choose what resonates with you about how much you want to drink on any occasion or whether to drink at all. To establish a positive mindset, you must identify your limiting beliefs and substitute them with empowering ones. We're going to show you how.

Our method is based on drawing a parallel between your bond with alcohol and a romantic relationship. In this book, for the sake of simplicity, we've given alcohol, "the lover," a more masculine personification. You can give your lover the gender, name, handle, image, etc., that works for you.

In your comfort zone with your charming and seductive lover, alcohol, everything in your life revolves around them. Whether you're happy, sad, or stressed out, you want to be with them—you want to drink. Your self-image and the image you portray to others are also linked to your lover.

We're going to help you to take a break from this attractive lover or even leave them forever. It will be difficult, but it's possible. After the initial shock has passed, you'll be able to see beyond your *denial* to how destructive this lover is. You may experience feelings of *anger*. You'll realize that *bargaining* keeps you in a state of avoidance and won't get or take you anywhere. Then comes the difficult part when you experience feelings of *depression,* because you realize that there's no common ground between you and your lover, and you need to make a decision. But as you keep going, there's a light at the end of the tunnel. As you begin *to accept* that you aren't going to return to your lover or take them back again, the destruction your drinking has provoked will be behind you.

We'll show you how not to get stuck in your *comfort zone* due to *limiting beliefs* and how to develop a *positive mindset* instead. This will enable you to face your fears and move through the *fear zone* and into the *learning zone*. Your positive mindset will develop quickly as you make new discoveries. You'll remember that *you're not a victim* and don't need to blame other people or circumstances. You'll be empowered to take responsibility for your own life and choices, and learn to use that power to explore new possibilities and make the changes you want.

Soon, you'll find yourself in the *growth zone*, with clarity of thought and awareness of your emotions and feelings, acting upon your good drives and intentions. You'll be in charge of your decisions regarding alcohol. *That seductive but destructive lover will no longer decide anything in your life for you.*

CHAPTER 4
YOUR COMFORT ZONE WITH ALCOHOL

"Spending time with my friends, with my people, at places that make me feel good, drinking my favorite wines, is something I love. I get out of my head and don't have to worry about anything. I love to be here, in this familiar space, feeling tipsy!" —Jessica

A comfort zone is a cozy place where we have a sense of safety, security, and protection. We have our familiar routines down pat, we have our preferred activities, we have our social circles. Everything feels known and controlled in this space, which makes it comfortable and extremely difficult to leave. But there's such a thing as being *too* comfortable. If there's no space to consider other possibilities, discover other realities, and grow, you can get stuck in your comfort zone—and *you are powerless there.*

In this comfort zone with your lover, your drinking, are all your limiting beliefs and a negative mindset. Your social circle of friends and peers pressuring you to continue drinking—even to the point of binge.

The societal conditioning you haven't questioned yet that normalizes and encourages drinking is another part of it. *These are all negative influences that you must change, as they keep you stuck in this unhealthy comfort zone.*

Let's start with the drink: It's always the same with this lover, but you're in a *state of denial*. You may *disagree* that your drinking is a problem or, at least, that the problem is a significant one. You say that you're not out of control. You're sure that eventually you'll get your drinking in check and enjoy it. You're not the only one convinced of this—the tenaciousness of this idea is shocking. In order to justify staying in your comfort zone, you try to find evidence that *there's no problem with your drinking.*

Then there are your *limiting beliefs*, which make you think that you're powerless to control your relationship with alcohol. Amidst other ideas, your limiting beliefs also keep you thinking that, without alcohol, you're shy and lame—not as cool, outgoing, relaxed, and fun as you'd like to be.

Your *mindset*, which is the attitude you have when facing obstacles and challenges, reflects that you're looking at your relationship with alcohol from a standpoint of loss—focusing on what *you won't have or what you could lose* if you reconsider your drinking—instead of potential gains. When your mindset is rigid or fixed, it closes you off to new possibilities in your life.

You may be questioning yourself (the *flash of clarity*) and losing self-confidence, but limiting beliefs and a negative mindset hold you back from changing. You may also consider that you "have to drink," to feel belonging with your social circle and not like an outsider.

At this point, you may feel like a *victim*. You keep finding yourself in difficult circumstances in connection with drinking, but you tell yourself that these consequences aren't your fault, they're out of your hands, and you're powerless to change. When you consistently drink in excess, you become an expert in playing the victim card and rationalizing a victim mentality.

> *"I had a big blowup with my best friend Rachel. I told her how low I've been feeling, and she asked me what I could try doing differently, like going for a walk after work to let off some steam, instead of straight to the pub. I felt that was really insensitive of her, like she's blaming me. She just doesn't understand how hard things are for me right now. My boss is so mean to me. It's not my fault. And alcohol helps me feel better." —Lorena*

Putting this altogether, your current situation with alcohol may include these elements:

- From a young age, you were told that one day you'd be able to enjoy all the "good things" that are linked to alcohol in our society. You're twenty-one or older, so it's time to enjoy your rights as an adult.
- Limiting beliefs connected to alcohol often stem from ideas you've had since you were a child, which your parents, extended family, and society around you have had a part in shaping. These beliefs hold you back from making progress.
- With a negative mindset, you feel that if you quit alcohol, you're going to lose something you enjoy: fun times, celebrations, friends, happy moments, and your cool drinking personality. Limiting beliefs combined with a negative mindset hold you back from growth.
- Your mindset is not only fixed but also has the characteristics of a *victim mentality*. This is characterized by feeling that you don't

need to change because it's not your responsibility and/or you're helpless to change—feelings of powerlessness and hopelessness.
- You may be scared about the uncertainty of drinking less or living alcohol free. This may be intimidating territory to explore, because if you don't have control of known situations, how much less power will you have regarding unknown ones?

Holding on to these factors sinks you deeper and deeper into your comfort zone, limiting your sense of possibility and hope for change. Without expanding your vision and trying new things to step out of your comfort zone, your self-esteem and self-confidence will shrink, and you may be limited in identifying and pursuing personal needs and goals. *Your lover will take the driver's seat of your life.* Gradually, this situation will deepen your belief that you aren't good enough on your own, that you *need* your lover, and so you keep crossing the line more and more.

In the next chapters we'll give you the tools to step outside this comfort zone and face the fears that pop up at this phase of your journey. Stay with it, and step by step, the road of life will open more and more to you. You're choosing to go toward a greater purpose: Experiencing your life to the fullest. Learning, growing, and feeling whole in constructing an exciting future that aligns with your truest desires.

Notes:

CHAPTER 5

THE COMFORT OF THE VICTIM MENTALITY

"Progress is happiness." —Tony Robbins

You may recognize that you're unhappy in your current comfort zone, whether physically, emotionally, or spiritually. If you cross the line consistently, you probably aren't growing and evolving. You're stuck in your comfort zone, neither seeing any progress, nor experiencing the consequent happiness.

In your comfort zone are various circumstances, people, and experiences over which you believe you have control. That control gives you a sense of power, but to maintain it, things in your comfort zone must remain the same, without changing. In fact, we may subconsciously reduce our world and possibilities to fit our limited comfort zone, in order to retain some (illusory) type of certainty. The nature of a comfort zone is that everything always continues in the same way; if something changes, it's perceived as a negative, a potential threat to the "comfort" of the comfort zone.

Although staying in your comfort zone can give you a sense of control, it also contributes to your feeling like a victim. We become comfortable with not taking responsibility or steps to move forward. Say, for instance, that you're drinking more today—who's to blame for this? Not you, and not your drink for sure. *It's your work, your kids, your partner, that friend! You deserve to drink.*

Tara, one of our clients, told us: *"Here's what I know: I don't have to change, this isn't my fault, and I don't have power over my environment. Bad things in my life are because of other people or situations."* Victims don't take personal responsibility; they either shame themselves, wallow in self-pity, make excuses, or accuse others. It's easy to feel like a victim regarding *your own* decision to drink.

Let's return to the concept of power. Since other people or situations are responsible for your behavior or troubles, they need to change, but not you; you don't have to change. You can continue doing the same things you've always done, *comfortable in your familiar world.* You're not to blame, because, as a victim, you're in the right, or you have a convenient excuse (rationalizing your actions). In general, people feel sorry for and sympathize with victims; nobody confronts or challenges them, so victims remain *passive.* Stepping out of your comfort zone and taking ownership looks really hard from this perspective, because a victim mentality disconnects you from your power.

Playing the victim *twists our perceptions of our reality and actions:*
- We reduce our world and possibilities to fit our limited comfort zone.
- We have a negative view of what is outside our comfort zone.
- We attribute problems and challenges entirely to other people or factors that we think are outside our control, disregarding that, for the most part, we do have some responsibility and power over our own actions and circumstances.

- We lose any desire to venture into other ways of being—learning new things and undertaking personal growth—which is self-destructive for our own potential and greatness.
- Our relationships are constantly in a state of tension, always focused on others' faults and who to blame, instead of using every opportunity to enjoy, nurture, and grow within others' presence.

Our lover, the drink, is partly responsible for keeping us stuck in this narrow comfort zone, preventing us from changing, blaming everybody and everything else, and making us cross the line more and more, as we get tangled in a vicious cycle of adverse circumstances and poor responses. Indeed, *the more you drink, the happier your lover is! But at what cost? How much is your lover taking from you? How much is your lover giving you?*

Notes:

CHAPTER 6
LIMITING BELIEFS KEEP YOU STUCK

Beliefs

Beliefs are the ideas we hold to be true about how we perceive ourself, others, the world, and how we interact. These views may be subconscious or unconscious, and so we may not be aware of them, but they feel certain and instinctual. We've accepted them as accurate for a long time, maybe from our early years; consequently, we see them as "real facts," valid and right, rather than just casual ideas that can be released or changed.

Our beliefs govern our lives, because they determine our mindset or attitude (positive or negative) regarding specific issues and our related thoughts and feelings. This, in turn, *determines our choices, decisions, and actions.*

When I, Alicia, was in first grade, my teacher told me that I was very good at math. She challenged me to do all the problem-solving exercises mentally without using a pencil, paper, or calculator. I did that for the whole year I was in her class, and I've continued to do math this way until now, because that teacher helped me to develop a positive mindset about doing math mentally. Whenever I need to make a calculation, I'm confident and positive. I do the math in my head. I act on impulse; I don't even think about it. I believe I can do it, and I act as if that belief is accurate.

Limiting Beliefs

A limiting belief is an idea that *confines us*, preventing us from taking action that can lead us to develop our highest potential. Here's an example of *limiting beliefs regarding alcohol.*

> *"I've been shy since I was little. I felt I didn't have anything funny or interesting to say, so people ignored me. My best friend was so outgoing and cool; she was always the center of attention. People followed her and laughed with her funny stories or comments. I always wanted to be like her, but the more I tried, the less interesting I seemed, and the less attention I received.*
>
> *"When I was a freshman in college, I was invited to a party. That was the first time I drank alcohol. It was only two beers, but I became exactly as I wished to be—funny, extroverted, and cheerful. While I was drinking, I felt popular. That feeling lasted all night. This was the beginning of my love story with alcohol. Drinking gives me the possibility of being who I want to be. I feel that I'll never be happy or attractive to others without a drink. I need the booze to be exactly the person I love to be."* —Annie

One of Annie's limiting beliefs is that drinking makes her a person she likes, the best version of herself. Her beliefs about herself and alcohol limit her from accessing or cultivating other resources. She could change her mindset and use different avenues to get the positives she thinks she gets from alcohol, but she's stuck. Annie's limiting beliefs have led her to make choices that are unhealthy for her and cause problems in her relationships and work, affecting her in the present and creating potential future consequences. She was unaware that her beliefs about "who she is" without alcohol were powerful enough to induce her to make wrong decisions.

Limiting beliefs regarding alcohol are critical because they determine:
- The attitude (mindset) we have regarding drinking, whether positive, negative, or neutral.
- The way we handle situations that involve alcohol. Limiting beliefs can impact the choices we make, which might lead to undesired consequences in the short and long term.

Is it possible to overcome limiting beliefs? Is it possible to switch each limiting belief into an empowering belief? The short answer is: Yes, it's possible!

What will your life be like when limiting beliefs don't control your thoughts and actions? To answer all these questions in more depth, you need to understand the beliefs that inhabit your subconscious mind, which influence your life and *keep you in a comfort zone with alcohol.* Limiting beliefs about alcohol prevent us from reaching our full potential and living our best life, because we have been misled to believe that *life without drinking is not fun, and/or that we aren't good enough without alcohol.*

Limiting beliefs are persuasive in some way or another and a type of self-imposed restriction that keeps you stuck. They're often formed early in life via many different sources, such as family, friends, and society in general. As children, we develop ideas based on our experiences, through the lens of what our family and teachers show us. In the beginning, these ideas are malleable and can change. However, with time, they become more accepted for the simple reason that we go into experiences based on our beliefs and wanting to prove the validity of what we feel. *We look for what we want to encounter*, because we want to be right and to confirm what we believe.

Many of these ideas about alcohol are ingrained in our culture, and consequently, *we accept them as valid*. For instance, if we see that there are alcoholic drinks at every party, we may assume that celebrating requires alcohol. Alcohol, therefore, becomes linked with happiness, accomplishments, and good times.

Our limiting beliefs—these thoughts about how we perceive the world and ourselves—guide our actions to the extent that they shape our lives. How does this happen? We accept these ideas as truths; from there, they *influence our choices and determine our actions*.

We may not be aware that limiting beliefs have such power, because *they come from the subconscious and take the form of impulses*. From that point forward, they create the confines of our life, becoming our reality, holding us back, leading to problems. The main issue is that limiting beliefs run on autopilot. We're not conscious of them, and they don't appear as red flags. *We act on impulses; we don't question them.*

The good news? These limiting beliefs are just in your mind. They're not backed by reality, and *you can change them*.

How can we discover and change our limiting beliefs? First, by *becoming aware of them*. Identify your limiting beliefs. Second, *take a closer look at the thoughts associated with each limiting belief*. As you excavate your past and what influences you, you may find what has created and supported these limiting beliefs about alcohol. Say you saw your parents cross the line with drinking every day; you may have developed limiting beliefs around alcohol, such as:

- Drinking every evening is normal.
- Since my parents drank regularly, I'm entitled to do it, too.
- Change is too hard once a path is set.

Chapter 6: Limiting Beliefs Keep You Stuck

Drinking Identity and Limiting Beliefs

Another way to think about our beliefs related to the self is to think about *identity*. *What does identity mean?* Identity is the core, the center, the foundation of the self. Our identity is who we think we are, how we think of and make sense of ourselves. We'd do anything to keep our identity consistent so that we feel aligned and in sync with ourselves.

Identity is the specific set of features that we can use to recognize and identify ourselves; it's how we perceive our self, including in comparison to others. It's part of how we develop our sense of place in the world. Identity informs how we present ourselves to others (or try), and how they perceive us, which loops back to inform or reaffirm our self-perception and presentation of who we are. An important part of what solidifies our sense of self is our perception of how *others* perceive us, what they expect of us, and how we try to tie in with that.

Identity plays a role in *motivation* and *action*. *To feel "right" or "whole" with ourselves, our identity, perceptions, and actions need to match up.* If a woman's identity is connected with *"I'm a good parent,"* she'll align her thoughts, feelings, and actions accordingly, always for the benefit of her children and family. If another woman's identity is primarily *"I'm fun and popular,"* she'll be at the center of parties and friend circles, up on the latest in pop culture and fashion, and have a social and outgoing personality.

In your relationship with alcohol, your identity may relate to your drinking habits: *"I'm a social drinker"*; *"I'm a solitary drinker"*; *"I drink with my girlfriends as part of the feminine drinking culture."* Some of *your motivations and subsequent actions—how you invest resources, time, and effort to match your motivation—will then stem from that identification.* Like a person who runs every day can think of herself as a runner, or a person who takes care of plants considers herself a gardener, a person whose pleasure centers around drinking and who puts time, energy, and money into alcoholic beverages and settings can be considered a "drinker."

"I realize that drinking has an important place in my life. Cocktails are an ever-present component during days off, evenings, weekends, vacations, time with friends, dates, celebrations, and holidays. As such, drinking is not only something I do but also part of who I am. The problem is that I don't know if I want to be identified as having this strong relationship with alcohol. Is that truly who I want to be? I'd rather be identified with other things" —Christine

You've probably heard about how alcohol changes people's personalities—how a person is one way when sober and "completely different" when alcohol is involved. Of course, a change like this escalates during binge drinking. The *typical "drinker" identity* is linked with the following:

- Always having an excuse to drink.
- Not sharing how much you normally drink, even with your doctors.
- Being aware of differences in your own personality—feeling that you're more social, relaxed, fun, and outgoing when you drink and different when you're sober (usually with a diminished sense of self).
- Thinking that drinking, by yourself or with others, is an essential part of adult life and a reward for completing your responsibilities—something *you "deserve."*
- Prioritizing drinks first. People, food, and other things come second when selecting where to go or what to do.
- Choosing events and activities based on having freedom to drink as much as you want; for example, at home, friends' houses, bars and restaurants, cruises, and all-inclusive resorts.
- Having a favorite glass and space at home for drinking.

- Spending time and money selecting, buying, and drinking alcohol; recycling bottles; and being surprised by the charges on your credit cards.

As you can see, a lot of *energy, time, and money* (our primary resources) go into enduring and maintaining your drinker identity. This doesn't even account for the resources that go into managing the psychological or physical problems and dependence that you're developing because of your drink. Your drinking identity can also affect your relationships, which in turn might cause you to drink more frequently or in greater quantities.

You should be aware that your drinking identity may be based on a collection of limiting beliefs about yourself and about connecting with others in conjunction with alcohol. In many ways, this awareness actually makes personal transformation easier, because if you can identify the limiting beliefs connected to your identity, you can better understand *what you want to focus on and change*. (Read more about building an alcohol-free identity in Chapter 17.) The next section will help you to identify your limiting beliefs about alcohol, yourself, and connecting with others.

Identify Your Limiting Beliefs about Alcohol

Following are the most common limiting beliefs about alcohol. Try to identify which ones are affecting you.

Limiting Beliefs Related to the Self
1. Everything in my life is connected to drinking. Change will be too hard. I'll never be happy again.

2. I like to drink because of how happy I am after my first two or three drinks and how extroverted I feel.
3. I just can't quit drinking; I've tried everything.
4. I'm not sure that I need to quit. I don't know if I have a problem with alcohol.
5. Being sober is terrible; who wants to be a "miserable sober"?
6. I'm afraid of not being successful at controlling my drinking or quitting alcohol.
7. I don't like to change. I love my life the way it is.
8. Drinking is in my culture. Tolerance for alcohol is in my genes. Everybody in my family drinks a lot. It's a way of life.
9. I'm more creative when I drink.
10. I love my personality when I drink.
11. I feel relaxed and stop worrying when I drink.

Limiting Beliefs Related to Connecting with Others

1. Drinking helps me connect better with others.
2. All the people who I hang out with drink a lot, and when we get together, we obviously drink. I can't change this.
3. My friends will judge my decision not to drink, and I'll be excluded.
4. I won't be able to meet new people or go on dates without having drinks. I'll be alone forever.
5. If I don't drink, people may think I'm an alcoholic or that I can't control myself.
6. I love to socialize and drink. I can't think of going to an event without alcohol.
7. I'm crossing the line at most of my social events, but it's okay since almost everyone else drinks a lot as well.

Chapter 6: Limiting Beliefs Keep You Stuck

Limiting Reliefs Related to Drinking

1. There are many aspects of drinking that I love, and I don't want to lose them. I enjoy trying different wines or beers. It would be boring to drink just water!
2. I love to end the day with wine. It allows me to slow down and connect with myself.
3. I feel good about my drinking routines when I am at home. I usually have a drink or two when I get home, another drink while I cook dinner, another drink when I'm on the phone, another drink when I eat dinner, another drink after dinner while watching TV.
4. Going out means "having drinks." I love to have drinks before, during, and after dinner. It gets expensive but it is part of the experience.
5. I'm a wine connoisseur and I get excited not only when I try new wines, but also when I revisit old ones. I love to cook and pair my favorite wines with food; it is so fun and such a relaxing experience that gives me knowledge about types of wine, regions, winemaking, notes, etc.
6. I like to try new cocktails often, either at good bars and restaurants or at home.

Change Your Mindset (Attitude) about Alcohol

Why make this change? The most important reason to change our mindset (attitude) regarding alcohol is because it's difficult to decide to change when we think we're going to lose or suffer as a result of that change; when we operate from a place of loss, based on limiting beliefs.

A practical step to help you reconsider your drinking is to make a list of all the seeming positives and negatives of alcohol and weigh them up. If you were to continue drinking without any change, the negative facts will outweigh any positives.

Instead of worrying that you're going to lose your lover, a source of comfort, the tool you use to connect with people, focus on how good you'll feel physically, how much money you'll save, the quality time you'll be able to spend with the people you love, and how much more productive and happy you'll be at home and at work. *Train your mind to focus on the positives of walking away from this lover.*

How can you make this change? We're going to give you the tools to help you change your limiting beliefs and positively shift your mindset to make a wiser choice. *The first step is to empower your mindset.* Let's create a positive starting point!

Think about this: You may be convinced that it's difficult to connect with others without drinking. But is that true? Think about the times after having a few drinks when you've had misunderstandings, arguments—even fights—with spouses, kids, extended family or friends. Holding on to the idea that we can't connect with people without alcohol is starting from a *place of loss.* If your mindset is negative ("I'm going to miss out!"), change is almost impossible.

An example of a positive starting point, beginning from a *place of winning,* is accepting the empowering belief that we can connect much better and more authentically when we're not under the undermining influence of alcohol. Without alcohol, we're less likely to experience self-inflicted negative situations, or to feel guilty or ashamed about things we've said and done.

Try It...
- Identify your limiting belief(s) regarding drinking. (You can use the lists in this chapter as an aid.)
- Make a list of all the seeming positives and negatives about drinking (or drinking as much as you do now), and weigh up these pros and cons.
- Choose one positive about reconsidering drinking to use as your empowering starting point.
- What's one action you can take based on your positive starting point?

Notes:

CHAPTER 7

THE NEGATIVE MINDSET THAT PREVENTS YOU FROM CHANGING

You now have a good idea about *what you might be losing currently, or what you stand to lose, if you keep drinking,* not only as far as your physical body and health but also when it comes to your mental health, positive sense of self-worth, and relationships with those around you—your family, friends, coworkers, etc. Enjoying progress and contentment in all these areas of your life is at risk *if you don't make a change.*

The first step to reconsidering your drinking is to set a positive mindset. *No decision can be made or maintained if we think that a choice will lead us to lose instead of gain in the long run.* A negative mindset will make it difficult, if not impossible, to change and make progress.

The key is to focus your mindset on *what you will gain* (not on what you *seem to be* losing) as you start distancing yourself from this lover and reduce your alcohol use. And remember, you're not alone in this situation: Alcohol is becoming a serious problem for a rising number of women in the US and many countries around the world.

Alcohol may affect us in two ways. The first is related to the problems and issues that can stem from alcohol, and the second is linked to what we fear will be taken from us if we reconsider drinking or become sober. There are many *inaccuracies and lies about alcohol* in our society, and these give rise to *erroneous beliefs;* for example, that drinking helps us to develop better relationships, that red wine is good for the heart, etc.

Alcohol never helps us. We don't gain anything from drinking; in fact, *we lose a lot.* Our purpose here is to help you to see what you're at risk of losing or ruining by continuing your current drinking pattern—be it your health, relationships, family harmony, life, work opportunities, and more.

We want you to fully recognize all the problems that alcohol brings into your life, but more importantly, to be aware of all the positive possibilities that will arise if you decide to reconsider your drinking. We can tell you from personal experience that an alcohol-free life is truly amazing!

Begin by shifting your mindset to see that, by deciding to drink with moderation or to quit alcohol, you *will win in big and small ways, in all aspects of your life, and this will improve your present and future.* Let this reality sink in for you. Accept what this expanded vision of success looks like. How does it make you feel?

Notes:

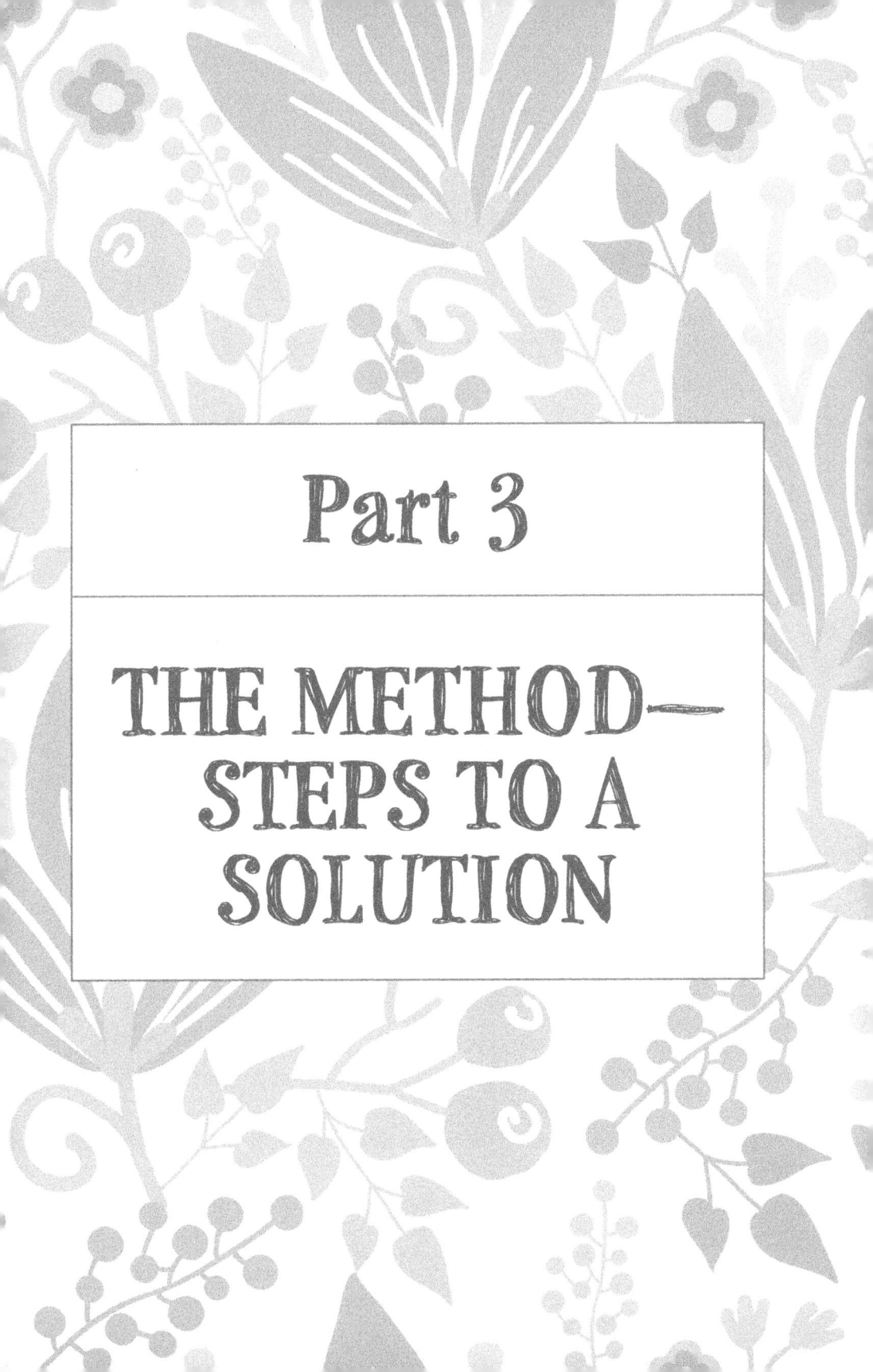
Part 3

THE METHOD— STEPS TO A SOLUTION

CHAPTER 8

WALK AWAY FROM THAT SEDUCTIVE BUT DESTRUCTIVE LOVER

If you could personify drinking and put a human face on this lover, what would they look like? Picture a lover who is *attractive and seductive but ultimately destructive.*

This lover has been invading your life, little by little, every day. At the beginning, they made their presence known from time to time when you were hanging out with friends. Then they started showing up during dates, dinners, and parties, taking up more and more space in your life. Now, they're with you every day. At any moment, whether you're out with others or at home, whether you're celebrating, relaxing, or coping with something—whatever is going on—*your lover is always with you.*

This lover is harmful and has the potential to damage you in many ways. They're selfish and self-centered; they don't care about you and your future. But because they're charming and captivating, they've taken the relationship between the two of you from casual to committed. Your lover is also your best friend and closest confidant. Maybe you're concerned that ending this relationship could be devastating, and you don't want to go through that. Your lover—your drink—is still *part of your comfort zone.* But deep down, *you know that this relationship is destructive, and that things will go wrong if you continue.*

"At the beginning of my involvement with alcohol, drinking was a social thing. I used to drink during get-togethers, parties, and some dinners at restaurants. Gradually, drinking became more important in my daily life.

"I need a drink when I'm happy, or depressed, restless, or bored. Whatever my state of mind, I want a drink. But not just one. I usually drink two, three, sometimes even four, glasses of wine—always keeping in mind that I need to moderate my drinking. I think, 'Today was complicated. I need a glass of wine to help me unwind,' but deep down, I know that it won't be just 'a glass' but several. Then I tell myself, 'I'll try to control it better tomorrow, for sure. I can try again tomorrow.'" —Rhonda

That "tomorrow" never arrives. The seductive lover remains *very close to you, convenient, and available.* Drinking is necessary today for one reason or another; tomorrow it will be for something else—until one day, you realize that alcohol is among the most important companions of your life.

Moreover, you begin to feel that you can't live without your lover. You *plan your schedule around your drinking.* You also ignore or excuse the numerous red flags popping up and don't pay attention to the other imperceptible (for now) ways alcohol disturbs your life. *Have you thought about that, how your drinking is troubling your life? What is it giving to you, and what is it taking away? What will happen in one year or five years from now? What will your life look like in ten years if you remain in this relationship?*

Chapter 8: Walk Away from That Seductive but Destructive Lover

At this point, the most vital decision you can make is to *break up with your lover*, for the following reasons:

- Gradually, you're becoming emotionally and maybe physically *dependent* on your lover, to the point where you need every part of your life to revolve around alcohol. You aren't your own independent person anymore; you need a drink in every situation you're in.
- This lover makes you feel *you aren't good enough*, that something is wrong with you since you're helpless to resist *their seduction.*
- Your lover *destroys your self-confidence.* All your promises to yourself to control your drinking are broken a few hours later, so how can you trust yourself?
- This lover *ruins your free days* with hangovers and feelings of regret, guilt, and shame.
- Your drinking *damages* your health, psychological well-being, relationships, finances, career, and future—*every part of your life.*
- There's *nothing new* for you to gain with that jerk. As you continue this relationship and become more emotionally dependent, there's no variety in your life; just the same drinking routines all the time. You progressively stop doing other activities since you have lower energy and fewer resources, and you may be more isolated than before.

Enough is enough! Why do you tolerate this? There's a sense of urgency here. You must think about yourself. This is your life, and you have only one. This lover isn't leading you to anything good—just the opposite, in fact. They're drawing you into a life controlled by dependence and limitations. For all these reasons and more, you should end this relationship, break up with your lover.

The interesting thing about this is: *You* must be the one to break up with your lover; they *won't break up with you*. Why? Right now, your lover is *taking everything from you*—your life, health, relationships, money, attention, and time—so there's no reason they'd break up with you. *You're the one who needs to end this relationship. Send this lover back home with all their stuff. Don't keep answering their texts or calls. Delete their number. Make this lover leave.* **Now**.

As you make the decision to start living free from alcohol, *you'll recover so much that you love—starting with your freedom—and find new things to enjoy.*

The Decision

A breakup implies *a decision* and *an action*. The most important (and challenging) part of breaking up with your drink is *the decision* to end the relationship. Lots of people spend years trying to take this step. As time goes by and they keep drinking, they may have *not only an emotional but also a physical dependence* on alcohol, which can require expensive and long treatments with a high risk of relapsing. Making the decision becomes more arduous as time passes because they become more and more dependent on alcohol.

Part of the difficulty of breaking up with your drink is that alcohol is the *most accessible, cheap, legal, socially accepted, and well-supported drug in the world.*

- *It's accessible and legal.* You can get alcoholic beverages in almost all restaurants, grocery or other stores, or gas stations. Sometimes you can even get drinks when you go to your hairdresser or nail salon or spend a day at a spa. You can drink at home. Absolute availability.

- *It's cheap.* There are all kinds of beverages at all sorts of prices.
- *It's socially accepted.* Alcohol is more than accepted, there's a kind of *social obligation* to drink. Choosing to be alcohol free might come with social stigma: that you've made this choice because you had an alcohol problem or can't control yourself. But drinking is well-supported.

So, how can we make this decision and act on our soundest interest? We must identify and work with both internal and external factors for this decision to become a reality.

Internal factors are your personal limiting beliefs (see Chapters 6 and 7) that have given you a false idea of reality and influenced your mindset. Remember that it's difficult to choose to change when we're operating from a place of fear or loss. Even though there are some short-term costs, the outcome and long-term gains are worth it. Remember your positive starting point. Reframe your decision to focus on the wins. For example, "I'm an alcohol-free woman living on my own terms" (versus thinking that without your drink you're "just another miserable sober").

External factors are linked to societal norms, social connections, and special events that traditionally include alcohol: everyday social life, vacations, holidays, celebrations, dating, etc. There's also a sociocultural norm that drinking is the way to get through difficulties. We cover external factors in more detail in Chapter 15.

As a result of making this decision and taking subsequent action to break up with alcohol, you'll become free of this destructive lover and open yourself to the future. You'll recover external and internal realities that were displaced by the influence of alcohol and regain your confidence and self-esteem in undoing the dependence.

Soon you'll have more positive resources—restored health, more free time, revitalized energy, better relationships, more productivity, and more money. You'll meet new, healthier people on this road. Life will improve, and after a while, *you won't feel like going back to your old habits and routines.*

Are you ready? The only things you need are a commitment and trust in yourself (and in us to guide you through) that you can *break up with that attractive, seductive, and destructive habit. Enough is enough. This is your life. It's time to move forward on your own.*

Try it...
- Make a list of the internal and external factors that make you drink.
- Clarify which internal and/or external factors are the *most dominant* in each situation (e.g., socially, at home, personal life, etc.) and—this is important—*when* they're holding you back. For instance:
    o "I drink during work happy hours to decompress from a long day and socialize with my colleagues."
    o "I drink with my girlfriends to connect better and feel that I belong to the group."
    o "I drink because I'm an introvert, and get-togethers make me anxious. With a couple of drinks, I feel at ease."
    o "I drink at night to stop my mind running; alcohol helps me to forget about my worries."

Breaking up with Alcohol and the Five Stages of Grief

In 1969, visionary Elisabeth Kubler-Ross outlined the stages that terminally ill people experience as they come to terms with illness and dying, which later became popularized as the *five stages of grief*: denial, anger,

Chapter 8: Walk Away from That Seductive but Destructive Lover

bargaining, depression, and acceptance.[43] Her findings were expanded to reflect the characteristics of *processing all types of personal losses*.

Looking at breaking up with alcohol as *ending an important relationship*, we use the framework of the five stages of grief to describe the experience and processes of letting go of this extremely negative habit. We're going to walk with you through this breakup.

The stages of grief don't always occur in chronological order. They can be skipped or revisited, sometimes without people's full realization until after the fact, and sometimes there's no way to avoid a certain stage. You may even feel like you're going through several stages at once. There's no set time frame for experiencing the stages of grief or working through all the feelings of this breakup. It's a process that can take days, weeks, or months.

It won't be easy to remove such an important part of your daily life and routine, especially if you've been in a central or committed relationship with alcohol. Your lover is taking so much from you that they want to remain close. They'll use all their seductiveness to convince you to stay, *to keep drinking*, making the process of letting go and grieving more complicated.

Acceptance, the fifth stage, may not be attained in a permanent way. It can be an ongoing experience, and we can move back and forth between the previous stages and acceptance. The good news is that, if we reach the acceptance stage, any reiterations we experience of the other stages will become easier and gentler than before, until they are no longer part of the journey.

For the sake of clarity, we'll present these stages—denial, anger, bargaining, depression, and acceptance—one by one.

---

43. Elisabeth Kubler-Ross and David Kessler, *On Grief and Grieving* (Simon and Schuster, 2014).

Denial

"I technically drink a lot, because I have a little bit of alcohol each day during the week and then multiple drinks when I go out on Fridays, but everything's okay. I've never experienced any severe consequences, like a DWI, getting fired from my job, or passing out in front of my kids. Those things could happen, but they haven't. I'm not an alcoholic, but some days are more difficult. If I have some problems with my kids, an argument with my husband, or something at work doesn't turn out okay, then this third drink is what I need. But it's not every day. Today is an exception. It's just this one time, and tomorrow I'll drink moderately.

"In the last few years, I've gone from drinking socially to drinking as a necessary part of my daily life. It's also something I keep secret from everybody, including me, to be honest. My usual feelings about my drinking are: (1) Today was rough; I need one more drink. I deserve it; I've earned it. (2) I don't want to worry about anything else right now; a couple of drinks will do the trick. I'll think about my problems tomorrow. (3) Today was great, I need to celebrate with a drink! (4) A drink makes any event more fun; I'll try not to cross the line." —Joyce

Denial is a losing battle. You feel you may be crossing the line here and there, but it's because of the other people or the situation. *Not you.* You still think you have *a grip on your drinking.* You tell yourself and others that you don't have an alcohol problem, that your drinking isn't out of control, or at least not to the point where it's noteworthy. Yes, that lover is still in your life, but they're not so bad; you're not going to be with them forever. Or maybe you think that you're still your own person; you don't depend on your lover. Everybody has a lover, and it's your right to have one, too.

These excuses mean that you can keep justifying how much you overdrink or disregarding the consequences, such as hangovers, relationship problems, and issues that you wouldn't have if you weren't drinking. You keep telling yourself that you don't have a problem—everybody you know drinks like you or even more.

There are *two beliefs* that people normally hold while in denial:
1. Alcohol isn't a problem, so talking about it is a waste of time.
2. If you don't have a major drinking issue, there's no point in taking a break or quitting.

There *comes* a point when *you can't keep denying your situation anymore*, and this will allow you to enter the anger stage. Frequently, people close to you will experience anger before you get to that stage: when they feel they can't tolerate the situation any longer, when they've had enough excuses from you, or when they don't see any positive changes. This anger can be positive or negative, depending on the type of relationship, degree of closeness, the style of communication used, and how scared they feel that you may be becoming an alcoholic.

Anger

"Lily asked me if I had a problem, and I answered immediately: 'What do you mean?' She said that lately I've been drinking way too much. I don't feel like that, but if I drink a lot occasionally, it's because of all the problems with my husband Dan. I can't trust him; he makes me feel so insecure. He's always in his world and doesn't seem to need me. Also, coming from the family I did, how can I not drink? Both of my parents passed out every single night! I have it in my genes, and, you know, it's impossible to go against what's in your blood." —Sally

Typically, anger is triggered when someone suggests that you might have a problem with alcohol. Their view may present *a significant threat to your denial.* You may feel upset if somebody assumes you can't control your drinking and are a borderline alcoholic. Your natural reaction is to lash out and blame their concerns on everybody and everything else, *not your dependence on alcohol.*

You can also experience anger if you feel you won't be able to drink as you normally do, leading to unpredictable personal and social consequences (for example, being considered a "miserable sober," feeling excluded or "missing out" on fun). The anger can be self-directed about needing to reconsider your relationship with alcohol, or if your overdrinking has created pain or problems for you or others. Anger can be directed to your loved ones, especially if they seem to have a different relationship with alcohol or be in a different stage on the journey.

Anger can be mixed with *fear,* because deep down you know that you've suffered, or will suffer, negative consequences if you continue drinking. Anger can also be muddled with *envy* of all those who can have a drink but are not dependent or never will be—those women who drink socially or for special moments only and then return to their everyday life without dependency.

Bargaining

"I know I'm drinking too much, but it loosens me up and makes me feel better about my job and with my family. Maybe I should try not to drink from Monday to Thursday, or perhaps white wine is better than red wine, or I could try vodka for a while. Also, if I devote some of my evenings to yoga or running, my restlessness may go away. But I want to make sure I can have my drinks at the end of the day, especially during the weekends. I need my wine. I can't imagine my life without it." —Lisa

Bargaining refers to thinking about and finding ways in which you can be with your lover in a more "acceptable" way—meaning, without being dependent, without their destructive possibilities. In other words, you're aware that you have a significant problem, but you're not ready to make the necessary changes to resolve the issue. You bargain with yourself as a way of trying to continue your relationship with your lover and still have some control.

For example, you may bargain to reduce your alcohol intake, have a "skinny drink," drink only on weekends or after 5:00 p.m., have a full glass of water in between drinks, avoid bingeing, or stay at events for a short time. Bargaining can go on and on—into infinity and beyond. But most of the time, bargaining doesn't result in long-term success, and the endeavor fails. The focus of bargaining is not on getting to the root of the problem and putting an end to it, but rather on trying to *avoid* trouble, please others, or "get by."

Bargaining can be useful in moving you closer toward a decision to be alcohol free. However, if you use it as an avoidance mechanism, the risk is that it could also keep you in your tiny, static comfort zone with alcohol for years, gradually leading you to becoming an alcoholic. Once you've reconsidered your drinking and decided to leave your lover, bargaining can be a risky technique that works against you on the long term. If you've decided to quit, bargaining with yourself can lead you to relapse.

Depression

"I'm less excited about going out with friends or on a date now that I've decided not to drink, so I've been making excuses or cancelling get-togethers for no reason other than my nondrinking. I know alcohol isn't good for me, but I wish I could drink the way I used to. I miss it. It's amazing all

the good things alcohol brings—fun moments, interesting conversations, enjoyable friendships, and romantic times. But because I crossed the line so many times, I can't have any of these anymore. I've become something I feared for a long time: sober but miserable." —Helen

At this point, you're definitely aware that being with your lover makes you unwell. Alcohol takes more than it gives you; *the negatives vastly surpass the positives.* You recognize your limitations. You aren't a "social drinker"; you're simply *crossing the line badly and frequently.*

On the other hand, living without your lover is hard! You know they're destructive, but their seductiveness still lingers and is overwhelming. Over and over, you ask yourself: *How am I going to live a good life and be happy staying sober?* You may think that sober people are cheerless, dull, and depressing.

You may feel caught between a rock and a hard place. You know how *destructive* alcohol has been and will be, but at this point, it takes *hard work and even suffering to let go of your drink.* This stage feels so hard, you might think, *I feel so bad, why should I take this path, or try to build new habits or engage in different activities, or meet new people? Is there any hope of feeling better?* You feel desolate, helpless, and hopeless. You want this change, to live without dependence on alcohol, and yet you may have feelings of regret, shame, and guilt for the damage your drink has caused you or how your addiction has harmed your loved ones' lives.

Acceptance

"Finally, I saw how my drinking was robbing me of opportunities. Gradually, I've been putting my life in order, including developing new routines, activities, and relationships. Now, I feel in control and like I

can improve my health. I abstain from drinking, and I've started a diet. I've already lost some weight, more than I have at any other time in my life. I feel great, full of energy. There's no more brain fog. There are many things I can do now because of the sense of discipline I've gained in being alcohol-free. I'm not battling myself anymore. I was sick and tired of the self-destructive path I was on for so long. I was suffering internally without real awareness of what was going on with me. Now, I have a sense of wholeness and clarity; my mood is calm. I feel empowered to do more, to try new things. I'm starting to understand more about myself and my loved ones. I know I'm at the beginning of my journey and that there will be temptations on the path. But I'm sure about this change. I embrace this way of life and accept myself, my past, and my decision to be alcohol free." —Beverly

Acceptance is a multilayered stage, and you may visit it more than once before you come to stay. It includes not only admitting (accepting) that you have a problem but also acknowledging (accepting) what your unavoidable fate will be if you don't reconsider drinking. It can also include accepting the new possibilities, growth, and relationships that becoming alcohol free will unlock for you.

Complete acceptance starts by acknowledging that you're in trouble, *taking decisive action to address the issue, and finally changing the situation.* Acceptance is an *active stage*, in which you're expected to take action to leave your drinking habit, which will improve your life.

The other part of the puzzle and the decision-making is to think about how you'll reconstruct your life without the negative influences of alcohol—what actions you're going to take *now* to heal and grow. If you've crossed the line for a long time, reconstruction may also include how you're going to repair damage caused to others.

The Action

Every heroine faces obstacles in their journey as well as opportunities to make a courageous step into the unknown. So far in your journey to reconsider your drinking, you've gained awareness of the societal norms that make drinking seem okay and yet that alcohol damages your health and well-being. You recognize the limits of your comfort zone with alcohol; the stagnation that comes from a victim mentality; and the limiting beliefs and negative mindsets, whether from internal or external factors, that keep you stuck. You understand that alcohol is a charming and seductive but ultimately destructive lover, and you've made the decision to end the relationship. You have the compass of the stages of grief to use in your journey.

Give yourself credit for being here, willing to take the plunge, to *make the break*. We applaud your courage. This is the time to pair your decision with a tangible action. Here's an opportunity for you to take a practical step that's daring and vulnerable and brave, something that responds to the truth within you about those flashes of clarity and your desire to live with freedom and authenticity.

The best way to act on your decision to leave your seductive but destructive lover is to *give yourself time away from your lover*. We suggest that you take at least twenty-one consecutive days without drinking. If you miss a day, that's okay. Just start the twenty-one days over again and keep going until you've had a full twenty-one consecutive days without alcohol.

These three weeks are both a challenge and a gift to your body and your health. Regardless of your long-term personal goal in reconsidering alcohol, taking a short break from drinking will help your body to readjust to your healthy baseline and build better habits. If your goal is to be alcohol free, you will be three weeks farther into the life you want. Ideally, we recommend that you give yourself at least three months of not drinking to firm up new habits, both physical and mental, and see a lifestyle change.[44]

Going through this part of the journey is tough and takes willpower, so practice self-compassion as you make this change. Every journey happens step by step. This one is no different. Take it one day at a time. Don't worry about tomorrow or the day after. Each moment, each hour, each day you get through is a step closer to living the life you desire. At the end of the twenty-one days (and certainly if you take the ninety days), you'll see that you no longer have the constant thoughts, craving, urges, and longing for alcohol that you suffered at the beginning.

You can take the action step of quitting drinking for twenty-one consecutive days right now or at any point ahead. Let's keep going!

---

44. The "21/90 rule" was first introduced by Dr. Maxwell Maltz in 1960. It's a practical idea for taking action that helps you to start with a smaller, more manageable unit of time (twenty-one days), working toward a longer time frame (ninety days) to create a lifestyle change.

Notes:

CHAPTER 9

LEAVE THE COMFORT ZONE AND VICTIM MENTALITY

If you've reached this chapter, you've already decided to reconsider alcohol (to either quit drinking or to drink in moderation), and you've started working on your mindset (your attitude). You've been honest with yourself: *Do I want to continue living this way, in this comfort zone with a seductive but conflicting and damaging partner?*

We've invited you to take an important personal step: *Officially calling it quits with alcohol and formally ending your relationship.* Whether your relationship was casual, central, or committed, you realized how far your drinking had taken you, and that *it was time to let it go.* That's a decision to leave your old comfort zone with alcohol. You're here because you want *a life of freedom from a habit that can turn into an addiction and ruin your life, health, relationships, weight, career, finances, and more.*

Leaving your comfort zone with drinking implies moving away from the habits you've built around drinking and even taking some time away from your drinking buddies. We're going to help you to step out of that limited comfort zone and away from your destructive, confusing lover. We respect your courage, and we're going to guide you through the process so that you can track your progress and accomplish the important goal you've established to live a better life for you and yours.

We ask you to keep an open mind and to work through each principle of our method. Don't shortchange yourself by skipping steps of the process. We assure you that this will work. Even if you've tried to take a break from alcohol before, this time it will work as intended. We know you can do this and that this is your moment. Right now! Not tomorrow, or next Monday, or right after the holidays. *Now is the time!*

When you make a decision and take action, you're opening a door to an unknown reality. There's nothing familiar about it, it can be uncomfortable and scary, but there's also some kind of magic in stepping into this uncertainty that will make you grow. What you can be sure of is that *you're the one who made this decision for you,* and that *you're going to do your best.*

Right now, you may feel a bit lost, like you're in unknown territory, and it's okay to feel this way. People decide to break up with alcohol and be sober or drink less for different reasons, because each of us is unique. It's important to create a *deep connection with yourself,* to renovate and come inside of *your emotional home, affirming your self-respect* for making this decision to live better. *Bring in compassion for your indecisions, doubts, mistakes, failures, and baby steps.*

What happened in your past is important because you're learning from that, especially from what hasn't gone well, the mistakes and missteps. We honor our past for where it's brought us, what we've learned, and the ways we've grown, but we *don't want to live in the past any longer.* We're going to learn about ourselves today, our patterns, why we drank, what triggers us to cross the line, and move forward with that information. Through this, we'll also learn and connect with our future potential. As the saying goes, *"Inhale the future, exhale the past."*

This time may be emotional and even frightening, but stay with yourself through these feelings. Root deeply into your authentic self, and be here, with what's real. You'll start having ideas and finding opportunities for how you wish to live your life, what you want to change, what you'd like to carry with you, and what must be left behind because it's not serving you anymore.

The last part of this exploration is to visualize a bright future:
- How do you want to live your life? Not what others want from you—just what *you* want.
- What step will you take today to match those expectations, change, and grow into this better version of yourself?

Keep walking away from that lover, from that tiny, limited comfort zone that's kept you feeling like a victim and not the winner you can be. This is going to be an exceptional journey for you as you think about what you truly want. As you move through life, free from the control of alcohol, take time to notice and appreciate your accomplishments, small and big. Each step is progress, and making progress is an excellent way to fuel happiness. *Let's do this!*

Notes:

CHAPTER 10

TRANSFORM LIMITING BELIEFS INTO EMPOWERING BELIEFS

Here's the one-million-dollar question: *How do we change our limiting beliefs about alcohol?* Forcing change or fighting against old ideas is unhelpful because it makes them grow stronger. As motivational speaker Tony Robbins says, "What we resist, persists.*" Instead, we can acknowledge the limiting beliefs and *build up new beliefs—empowering, transforming beliefs this time—to take the place of the old limiting ones.*

Following are the most common limiting beliefs about alcohol regarding the self, connecting with others, and drinking as a social activity. We also present the empowering beliefs you can use to replace old thinking and lay the foundation for a positive mindset.

Putting these empowering beliefs together illustrates *how great life looks when alcohol is out of the picture*—a vision that can help us get to the other side of this change. Use this information to help you shore up your change to reconsider your drinking or move you closer to taking that step, in conjunction with caring for yourself through the five stages of grief.

---

* Robbins, Anthony. UPW Event. Robbins Research International, Inc.

Limiting Beliefs about the Self

1. Limiting Belief: All my life is connected to drinking; change will be too hard. I'll never be happy again.
"Whether I'm stressed out, lonely, or bored, I have to start my evening with a glass of wine. It helps me cope with my divorce. It alleviates pressure about work and finances since I have my salary only on which to survive. Alcohol has also helped me to look more extroverted, fun, and interesting on the few dates I've had lately. My 'wine time' is a time to let everything go and have a good moment, even on difficult days. But when I wake up the following day, I don't feel well, with a hangover or something that makes the night before not as relaxing as I'd hoped—and I still have the same challenges! Sometimes I question my drinking, but after 5:00 p.m., I forget about that. I feel good for a couple of hours, and later I'm tired, but I keep drinking. I go to sleep, wake up, and everything starts again. This is my life." —Gabrielle

By continuing with your same level of drinking, you're limiting your life to your small comfort zone. This isn't the best option available to you. Your life is more than this tiny space that prevents you from changing, growing, and making progress. You won't reach your fullest potential if you're stuck in your comfort zone and numbed by the effects of alcohol.

- *Empowering Belief: If I choose to take a new step outside my comfort zone, it's inevitable that I'll feel some discomfort and need to face my fears, but it will get easier with practice.*

Chapter 10: Transform Limiting Beliefs into Empowering Beliefs

Your steps will become stronger as you cross the learning zone and move to the exciting growth zone. You'll find many new possibilities there. As your energy and vitality are restored, you'll feel better, with increased desire and energy to explore those exciting new options.

2. Limiting Belief: I like to drink because of the joy I feel.

"When I have a drink in my hand, I feel happy. This is why I love to drink. I feel good in the lead-up to drinking, the anticipation, and with the first sips. It's true that I may become a mess afterward, but I love that first part. The morning after is another story." —Lucy

You probably do feel happy while on your first or second drink, but most people feel low or numb afterwards. (Of course, there are exceptions; some people might feel happy and energized all night, and other factors can play into this, like social cues.) But since alcohol is a depressant, it naturally lowers motivation, joy, and pleasure. You may also experience low energy on the morning after, including a hangover with all the ugly symptoms that brings. *Not joyful at all!*

- ***Empowering Belief: When I take a break from drinking, my nervous system will adjust and get healthier.***

In comparison to using alcohol, people report having less brain fog, fatigue, depression, anxiety, boredom, and dullness when they reduce or stop drinking. On the other hand, alcohol-free people feel more relaxed, calm, and in balance than when they were drinking.

3. Limiting Belief: I just can't quit drinking.

"I see that there are people who can drink in moderation or who have decided to become alcohol free. I can't do that. I think I'm differ-

ent. *For some reason, I can't quit or become only a social drinker. What's wrong with me?"* —Meredith

This limiting belief shows that you're *stuck in your comfort zone.* You've concluded that you can't quit, because you haven't been able to do it before, or because other people you know weren't able to quit or reduce their drinking. You may be afraid of everything outside your lifestyle and routine, but your current way of life with alcohol represents only a *minimal part of your potential reality.*

- **Empowering Belief: Everybody can change—including me!**

Consciously or subconsciously, *we are all changing all the time.* Making this positive change to leave your relationship with alcohol starts with *believing you can change.* It also includes adjusting your mindset, identifying and facing your fears, taking action, and learning how to live differently. This will allow you to go outside your comfort zone, and your life will enter another dimension.

4. Limiting Belief: I'm not sure that I need to quit. I'm not convinced I have a problem with alcohol.

"I'm doing so well in my job, I'm a good mother, I have a fulfilling marriage, I think I'm fun and social. Sometimes, when I drink too much, I feel that I'm not in control and that reducing my drinking is beyond my power. Nevertheless, since nobody says anything about it—because they drink like me—I keep going as though all is well. I'm not sure if I have a problem with alcohol, so I have no clue what to do. It seems like things are good enough." —Sharon

There are two main ways in which alcohol dependence can affect people:

1. *Physically*: People with Alcohol Use Disorder may experience strong cravings and physical withdrawal symptoms. Therefore, they need to keep drinking to function at their normal level.
   o Some people have a physical dependency but also have developed a high tolerance, which makes them a *high-functioning alcoholic*.
2. *Emotionally or psychologically*: People who are constantly thinking about their next drink but don't seem to experience physical symptoms or serious consequences yet.

It doesn't matter if you're addicted or not. *If you aren't yet, you may become addicted in the future*. It could be just a matter of time because alcohol is addictive.

- ***Empowering Belief: What matters is the quality of my life. Is my drinking improving my life now and for the future?***

Be honest with your response, since acknowledgement is key to addressing what's not going well. When a decision is in our best interests, it's smart to make that choice sooner than later. That way, we increase the positives and reduce the negatives in the short and long term. It's never too late to take a step in the right direction. If you're not sure whether you need to quit, take a break for three months and see what happens and how you feel.

5. Limiting Belief: Being sober is terrible.

For many people, being sober equals being miserable. Our cultural environment, friends, and family may suggest that drinking less or being alcohol free implies that you're missing out on the fun, that you or your life are boring, or that you're doomed to be stressed out.

"The first thing people ask when somebody doesn't drink is if that person is a former alcoholic. Another stereotype is that the person is boring, that you're dull and miserable if you don't drink. There's a kind of intimate friendship that's based on drinking together and sharing vulnerable feelings while drinking. I feel this type of relationship takes a lot more time to develop with somebody who's sober. Sobriety makes you look different—unattractive or less fun in some way. Some people who drink in excess are uncomfortable and freak out if you say you're sober. They think you're stuck-up. They expect you to drink with them and not judge how much they drink." —Hayley

- **Empowering Belief: I'm upgrading, not downgrading, my life; everything will be more beautiful, whole, and happy without drinking.**

This is an opportunity to go beyond stereotypes and envision yourself without the limitations of alcohol. *Who are you? Who were you before you started drinking like this?* And most importantly, *who can you become in this new future?*

6. Limiting Belief: I'm afraid of not being successful at moderating or quitting my drinking. I've failed many times before.

"I know that I should quit or moderate my drinking. But I've tried before and it didn't work. I'm afraid that this will be another failure. Then I'll have to face that I'm not good enough, that I couldn't quit, that I'm not effective at looking out for what's best for myself or honoring promises to my spouse and family." —Donna

Success in quitting comes not because we don't fail, but *because we do fail at times (we're human), we learn from that, and we get up, learn the lesson, build a strategy and try again.*

- ***Empowering Belief: When I fail or face a challenge, I can use the experience to** ask new and better questions, to try new things, and I'll evolve.*

We grow based on what we learn when we fail or make mistakes. This time of learning is about us, our routines, what works or doesn't work. Think about this as a trial-and-error process: *Use what works, and discard what doesn't.* You're going to come through this with different ways of dealing not only with alcohol but also other challenges in life. We're giving you the tools you need, so approach this time with confidence that it *will* be different. Align your mindset to a position where you're sure you will win. *And remember, if you follow this method, step by step, success will be inevitable.*

7. Limiting Belief: I don't like to change because I'm in my cozy comfort zone. I love my life the way it is.

"I'm functioning normally in most aspects of my life. As long as I can maintain my job and spend time with my family, there's no problem with my drinking. I need it at the end of the day. I'm affected by several problems and am constantly juggling so many things. Why do I have to change? I need a drink, and I deserve it." —Elaina

Change is the only constant we have in life, and it's a force for good. Change can definitely be uncomfortable, but as grownups, we have the capacity to do things we *need* to even when we don't *want* to. Ignoring the need to change or opting to do nothing about it when you may be entering into an addictive habit is like burying your head in the sand. Use other motivations (health, independence, longevity, practicing courage, etc.) to get you going. Don't let fear stop you. Believe that you can change—everybody can! The number one characteristic of human beings is their *capacity to change and adapt*. Change is difficult, but being idle is worse.

- ***Empowering Belief: My whole life will improve when I go outside this small comfort zone!***
Face your fears and get going anyway, applying what you've learned here. Get curious and dig into why you don't like to change. Ask yourself: *Where does the resistance to this change come from? What is this about?* Finding the courage to change will improve your self-esteem and confidence, which are the *motors of the self.*

8. Limiting Belief: Drinking is in my genes; everybody in my family drinks a lot. It's a way of life, part of my culture.

"*Drinking is in my true nature. I come from a family where alcohol was part of everything—the good, the happy, the difficult, the problems. If we had a celebration, a funeral, or anything in between, there were always drinks. There was a lot of overdrinking, but nobody was considered an alcoholic. All I know is what I learned from my family.*" —Renee

According to several studies, only part of the predisposition to drinking is related to genetic conditions. In addition, we can become conscious of familial or societal factors that play into a habit and choose to think or act differently. We don't have to be influenced by those factors—or at least not to the point where we give up critical thinking and decision-making power and act on autopilot.

- ***Empowering Belief: I can make personal choices that are better for me and different from the family patterns and routines I've observed, learned, or inherited.***

Chapter 10: Transform Limiting Beliefs into Empowering Beliefs

There are many ways to live, which can lead to a range of positive or negative paths. You have the power to decide for your life. Your determination to change can also become a positive example for your family.

9. Limiting Belief: I'm more creative when I drink.

"When I drink, I feel more inspired, but I do things I didn't plan—even things I told myself I wasn't going to do—or I say ridiculous things. Sometimes I think I'm creative, but occasionally I feel that I'm behaving like an idiot or, actually, like a drunk person. Sometimes I feel I have to be funny, and I go beyond what's appropriate. The next day I feel embarrassed by myself and the consequences I've created, especially when it bleeds into interpersonal issues. In those moments, I ask myself why I do this." —Caroline

Because alcohol is a depressant and affects your physical and mental state, it affects your creativity, too. You may feel you're more creative when you drink, but we invite you to question if this is true. Make note of when you're the most inspired and invigorated, and analyze your findings. In our opinion, this state happens when you're relaxed and have an open, sharp mind. This is more likely to be the case when you're sober and focused versus experiencing brain fog.

- ***Empowering Belief: When I liberate and clear my mental and physical potentials, many creative means will open to possibilities I haven't discovered or even considered yet.***

Limiting Beliefs about Connecting with Others

1. Limiting Belief: Drinking gives me a better connection with others.

"Meeting up with my girlfriends means drinking together. Alcohol has such a central role in our circle that if I don't drink, there will be a wall between me and some of them. They may feel judged; they may judge me or make me feel like I don't belong to the group. Drinking is seen as 'normal behavior,' and if you don't drink, you should have a good explanation, like, 'I'm on antibiotics,' 'I'm on a diet.'" —Riley

Many people drink convinced that alcohol facilitates their connection with others when often it does the opposite. Drinking may smooth relations during the first or second drink, but if you continue drinking, rather than creating a better connection, you're opening the door to negative consequences and conflict.

- *Empowering Belief: Without alcohol, I'm less likely to feel guilty or ashamed about what I've said or done. I'll be operating at a high level of connection.*

When not under the invalidating, impulsive influence of alcohol, you'll relate to others better. There's a stronger possibility of developing real friendships beyond having just alcohol in common.

2. Limiting Belief: I won't be included in my group. My friends will judge my decision and reject me or refuse to hang out with me. I'll be an outsider.

"With my friends, if you don't drink, you don't get invited; you're not part of good conversations and jokes. It's like you're an outsider, the

person who challenges party norms, the one who embarrasses the rest of the group. They think they can't trust you. Being included is important. So instead of allowing yourself to be mocked or excluded by your friends, you go ahead and drink." —Geraldine

"There's a peer pressure that includes judgment if you don't drink. Besides, nobody wants to hang out with you—it's like you're not part of the group. There's an attitude of, 'If you don't drink, we can't trust you.' So, you drink to belong. The more you drink, the more you preserve the friendships with those who drink, and the opposite: when you don't drink, they may judge you, and they don't invite you anymore." —Mayra

If your friends are all drinking buddies, they will try to sabotage your plan to quit or drink less, or they may disconnect from you *until you're "normal" again, meaning you're drinking with them.* These people are unlikely to encourage and support you to reconsider your drinking or move toward being alcohol free. The truth is that some people won't accept or like us when we're sober. This is a challenging and sometimes painful reality, because being connected with others and belonging is an important need for all of us.

- ***Empowering Belief: Without the negative influence of alcohol, my best self will show up and shine without the harmful effects of being tipsy or worse.***

Yes, you may find that you don't fit in anymore with groups that use alcohol to connect and spend time together. With time, you'll find new friendships, new groups linked to your alcohol-free lifestyle that will be more fulfilling than before. True friends will see in you someone who makes positive decisions and acts accordingly. They'll stay friends because they value who you are, whether you drink sometimes or not at all, and empower you to live better. People who judge and abandon you for reconsidering your drinking aren't worthy of your friendship. You'll find new relationships and tribes while on this constructive path of your life.

3. Limiting Belief: I'm single, and without having drinks, I won't be able to date. I'll be on my own forever.

"Dating can be hard since people may make up their minds about you based on whether you drink and think you're boring if you don't. Besides, where do you go on dates? Obviously, to restaurants and bars! The problem doesn't end with your being alcohol free. The other part is that it can be hard to socialize with someone who drinks a lot. So, the problem goes two ways." —Joanna

Drinks can be an important part of the dating scene. There may be a sense of expectation to have a couple of drinks during your first meetup (or first few dates). It's a dating norm in many ways. If you decline a drink, you may feel you have to explain why, and you might not be ready for that.

Another factor is the stigma of being sober. The other person may think that you're a recovering alcoholic or that you can't control yourself with alcohol. Nobody wants to feel judged or labeled while trying to make a good first impression.

- ***Empowering Belief: When I'm true to myself, I'll have more authentic communications and interactions on dates versus creating a false image of myself because of the adverse effects of alcohol.***

Chapter 10: Transform Limiting Beliefs into Empowering Beliefs

You always have the option to date other sober people, to not drink, or have a nonalcoholic beverage on dates. If you chose to date people who drink, be aware that some people won't be comfortable with your being sober. If that's the case, they may not be a potential longer-term companion since their lifestyle is different from yours. Holding to your convictions in dating can provide a good filter and prevent future relational problems.

Limiting Beliefs about Drinking

1. Limiting Belief: I love some aspects of drinking, and I don't want to lose them.

"There are some things I love about drinking: how a simple gathering becomes a party, how I can connect with people in a deeper, more intimate, fun way. I don't think I'm going to have these benefits without drinking." —Cheryl

The reality is that the negative parts of drinking surpass any positives it can have.

- ***Empowering Belief: I'll be winning, not losing, by going without alcohol.***

There's nothing alcohol gives that's *not available through other means.* That's right! Read it again!

2. Limiting Belief: I'm crossing the line at most social events, but it's okay since almost everyone else is overdrinking as well.

"I usually drink a lot, but I'm not the only one. I'm not even the worst one. Frankly, if you don't drink, you don't have fun. You don't make 'real friends' without alcohol. Cocktails and wine bring people together. Life is

complex, and I think we deserve those moments when we can chat, laugh, and relax without inhibitions. In my social circles, everybody overdrinks, but since we're all on the same page, it doesn't feel like we're doing something wrong. We can't all be alcoholics, right?" —Laura

Your drinking may not get the attention of others, and it might be "normal" by your current social standards, but does that mean it's completely okay? Comparing yourself with people who drink as much as you or even more doesn't give you a clear indication of how you're doing in this area.

- ***Empowering Belief: Alcohol is highly addictive. If I keep drinking in the same way, this habit can worsen or become an addiction.***

Drinking in excess is a negative factor in your life. At worst, alcohol causes you to lose ground and saps your energy, vitality, and health, becoming a deeply entrenched addiction. At best, staying with alcohol will keep you static, with fewer positive options and opportunities as time goes by.

You don't have to let alcohol be stronger than you. You can resist these urges and create balance by taking a break from alcohol and focusing on you as you continue following the steps in this book.

In conclusion, if you used to cross the line, maybe you haven't seen any red flags yet, but you've been *fighting yourself and trying to moderate your drinking for years*. You might not be drinking every day, you might not day drink or binge drink, but you *always want another drink, and drinking is on your mind most of the time*. You might also experience frustration, shame, guilt, and a loss of self-confidence, because you haven't been able to follow through with what you've decided to do.

Chapter 10: Transform Limiting Beliefs into Empowering Beliefs

When we become emotionally dependent on alcohol, gradually we build our identity around our drinking: the booze we like, when we want to drink, the people we want to drink with, the places we go to have drinks, and so on. We think that drinking defines us and determines an important part of our routines, and so it becomes an *ever-present factor* of life. More importantly, we feel *powerless to change this situation.*

We must make a change in our identity. We don't have to force this change or fight against our limiting beliefs, because this increases our focus on the problem, and it intensifies resistance, making those beliefs stronger. But we should identify and acknowledge our limiting beliefs. Then we can reframe and center our attention on positive, empowering beliefs about those same issues and build new mental connections for how we think of ourselves and social situations in relation to alcohol. By doing this, we change our mindset and move past the way we used to feel about drinking. We start to build a solid foundation that will empower us to go forward instead of limiting our potential. It's a *total life transformation!*

It's *a choice* to switch your focus from limiting to empowering beliefs. This is something you must decide for yourself. You're the one with the control and power over your approach.

We want you to see and think of yourself as the *product* of your empowering beliefs rather than the *consequence* of your limiting beliefs. And now *you have a new identity on which to build your realities—an alcohol-free queen!*

This powerful stage is more than just *"not drinking."* It's going outside the tiny comfort zone you had with alcohol that blocked you from seeing your true reality and potential and acting positively. It means facing your fears, moving past them, and building a new reality with what you've learned. Consequently, you will promote *growth and transformation in yourself.*

Growth implies progress, and we know that progress equals happiness for the majority of us, and this is precisely what alcohol slowly takes away. What you had before was *regression and a loss of your identity to a beverage that kept you small, numb and contained.*

Your decisions are in your hands now, and this makes you *own yourself.* Use your newly awakened consciousness, self-empowerment, and ownership of your decisions to create a life of freedom, health, energy, vitality, productivity, and joy.

Now, without your drink, you can build your life exactly as you want it to be.

Try it...

1. Identify your limiting belief(s) regarding drinking and the empowering belief you'll focus on instead. You can use the list in this chapter as a guide or adapt your own.
2. Tell yourself in a peaceful way, with kindness, respect, and self-compassion:

    1. I no longer accept the limiting belief that:
    - *The reality for me going ahead is:*

    2. I no longer accept the limiting belief that:
    - *The reality for me going ahead is:*

    3. I no longer accept the limiting belief that:
    - *The reality for me going ahead is:*

3. Repeat to yourself the points you've written down when you awake in the morning, during moments of reflection throughout the day, and as the last guided thought at night (to take it to a subconscious level).

Notes:

CHAPTER 11

PRACTICE A POSITIVE MINDSET

Practicing a positive mindset is key to orienting your mind and actions for success. You've decided to quit drinking or to drink in moderation, and *you're going to do it*. This will be your accomplishment, and you're about to create a plan for total success. *Picture yourself winning*!

During this process, you've been realizing that you can be the creator of your own life by taking charge of yourself and making choices that are aligned with reaching your full potential. Remember, *nothing significant is going to be lost, and everything will become better. Repeat this*. What's important now is to embrace uncertainty, get out of your comfort zone, and trust that you're making the right decision.

Now you must consider the following to develop and maintain a positive mindset:
- Look at alcohol differently by directing your attention to the factual downsides of drinking and how much it was taking from you, rather than to what you may have been conditioned to believe about the "positives" of alcohol.

- Become informed of the effects of alcohol consumption and strengthen your decisions based on that awareness.
- Create new habits for success by engaging in or avoiding certain situations. For example, instead of staying in or going out to drink, go to the gym, take a late afternoon or evening yoga or workout class solo or with friends; wake up earlier in the morning to do something you enjoy versus staying up late drinking the night before.
- Generate a system to track your progress, making a step toward your goals as frequently as possible. It's difficult to change what you don't measure. It's important to keep evaluating your progress and analyzing the situations and/or people that lead you to drink, with the purpose of making plans to avoid those situations and go in another direction.
- Reflect on your actions and their consequences. Learn how to change directions when your steps or outcomes are not in line with your goal.
- Anticipate difficult situations and plan ahead for how you can manage or exit the situation.
- Practice being kind to yourself when you mess up. Maybe you've made a mistake, but this doesn't define you. What can you learn from what happened, and what can you do differently next time around?
- End each day with recognition of your accomplishments, lessons learned, and a few focused to-dos for the next day.

Following is some skin on how to apply these steps toward building a positive mindset.

1. How to look at alcohol differently: Consider the actual consequences of drinking. Your worldview of alcohol and drinking may be based on personal experience and the experiences of those around you.

This is a *partial representation of reality* and is likely to be overly optimistic, especially given cultural messaging and norms about alcohol. Expand your view and make it more fact-based by reading up or watching documentaries on the topic to better understand other realities that you may have overlooked or underestimated.

Through these other sources of information, you'll find stories of people like you, successful people who started drinking in the usual way—socially, in their personal life, as part of their culture, etc.—and in a few years, became alcoholics. People who have *developed an addiction*, often reaching a point of no return, started just like you, but they lost control *without realizing it*. They're unhappy, they wish they'd never started drinking, and they regret not doing anything sooner when it may have been easier to control their dependence and to change. Put yourself in their shoes and imagine where you could end up if you don't change. Then imagine what could be different by taking even one small step today toward your vision of winning.

2. Analyze your limiting beliefs about alcohol: Using the information from Chapters 6 and 10, look at your limiting beliefs more closely. Remember that limiting beliefs are a harmful, damaging influence, and it's impossible to make a change when your mindset (attitude) is in a negative state—feeling that you're going to lose or focusing on what you can't do, instead of how much you're going to gain and the new things you could enjoy as a result of changing.

The following are examples of why you must let go of your limiting beliefs about alcohol:

- *"I'm under so much pressure, and drinking is the only thing that gives me relief."*

If you're in the middle of stressful situations or dealing with difficult people, drinking will actually complicate the situation even more. Your clarity and coping mechanisms will be diminished. Because alcohol lowers inhibitions, this can add more negative elements to an already challenging situation. The result is that *you'll have more pressures and stress—not less.*

- *"Drinking helps me to be more socially confident."*

What you're really looking for is that sudden surge in confidence that, for some people, is linked to the first or second drink. Past that and with more alcohol, that feeling evaporates and we're no longer presenting our best self. When you're tipsy, you can *think* you're being fun and outgoing, but you might actually become vulgar, repetitive, and disrespectful without realizing it.

- *"Drinking is fun; it's a happy lift."*

In our culture, alcohol not only prevails in daily life but is significantly associated with celebrating. From there, *it's easy to wrongly assume that alcohol equals happiness and joy.* Connected with this limiting belief is the tradition of toasting, raising a glass, to honor someone or something. What really lifts our minds and emotions are the people, activities, events, and interactions we're commemorating. *Alcohol is a depressant* and acts very strongly to suppress the fun and happiness we may be experiencing.

- *"Drinking helps me release my worries and calm down."*

Drinking doesn't resolve any of your problems and *adds another worry* to the ones you already have. This is a serious concern since alcohol is addictive, and after a while, it becomes harder and harder to reconsider or quit drinking. Now you still have a choice, but it's a small window of opportunity. Alcohol can add new problems to situations and relationships, and that's not counting the harm it does to your body and well-being. So, this is the time to break up with alcohol. By doing this, you're transforming your life!

Notes:

CHAPTER 12

CONQUER THE FEAR ZONE

We trust that you're still with us on this adventure of leaving your comfort zone with alcohol, that you're questioning how much you drink and your routines around drinking. Step by step, you're growing, you're evolving. This is an essential part of the human experience, and we admire your perseverance. It's also incredibly human and inevitable to experience fears—we all have them. *Growth and fear go hand in hand* when we refuse to let fear hold us back from progressing toward our goals and use fear as a cue of what to pay attention to and act on.

In this chapter, we're going to talk about facing fear of change and fear of the unknown and help you to discover facts about yourself that maybe you haven't noticed before. You'll be able to set a goal, manage new situations easily, and see your self-esteem growing in the process. These positives will boost your self-confidence for future goals and new life adventures.

"I started drinking when I was twenty-four. I met my husband one year before that. I thought he was the man of my dreams, and he was, at least for some years. Life got busy between my husband, the birth of our first daughter, my job, and spending time with a group of girlfriends.

We would discuss every topic imaginable, from politics to fashion. My drinking went from entertaining social drinking to much farther than okay. As my drinking progressed, I started drinking by myself.

"Every part of my life revolves around alcohol now, whether I'm with friends or my husband, or just by myself, and I always have more drinks than expected. I keep telling myself that tomorrow I'll do better, I'll have just two drinks and be done for the day. But tomorrow becomes today, and the same thing happens again. I can see that I'm trapped between the anticipation of drinking and crossing the line badly, and I'm using events, people, or circumstances as excuses to drink. This is my life today: stuck and unhappy, but I can't tolerate the idea of not having a drink again, I will lose out on all the fun, relaxation and socialization." —Suzanne

"When I get to the end of the day or the weekend, I feel that I need a drink. Everybody around me drinks like me or even more. I'm aware that drinking like this isn't a good fit for my career and lifestyle. Now that I am divorced, I wish I could feel more confident to date again and find a long-term relationship. Instead of drinking less, I eat less than before, just the bare minimum. The alcohol hits me differently—badly, often—since I'm drinking on an almost empty stomach. My self-esteem feels extremely low because I can't reduce or quit my drinking. This also makes it difficult for me to lose weight and see progress with my other goals. I feel stuck and intensely hopeless." —Mary

Suzanne and Mary are still in their fear zone. Once you take steps to leave the comfort zone you have with alcohol, the challenge that awaits you is crossing the challenging fear zone in order to reach the zones of learning and growth. We'll provide you with information to help you get through this fear zone with success.

To start, here are three steps you must practice and keep coming back to:

1. *Connect with your positive mindset,* believing that *your capabilities will expand according to your needs.* Stay positive during the process, even during uncomfortable times.
2. *Become aware of resources and insights* that can help you in confronting your fears. For instance, think about something difficult you've overcome, or a flash of clarity about your future if you keep drinking like this. In addition, connect with your emotional home through meditation, yoga, or with the simplicity of a moment of silence and solitude.
3. *Use your feelings of fear in a positive way.* We're more perceptive and alert when we're frightened or scared, so we're more ready to take action. Fear prepares us to react to new situations—so feel the fear and use it as a positive cue to change. Bring your fears into play to move forward.

When you're leaving your comfort zone with your drink, what *you really fear is the unknown.* You're leaving behind the day-to-day routines you're used to, where everything is the same and *feels* like it's under your control. *Your comfort zone is an easy, cozy place, but it lacks challenges or opportunities for growth.* Nobody progresses while they're stuck in their comfort zone. Indeed, the prevailing feeling there is *comfy but trapped.*

Going through the fear zone can be frightening and challenging—that's what prevents most people from breaking up with alcohol, because this is the place where *uncertainty is powerful.* We don't know what we'll find, and we may wonder if we'll have the necessary resources to deal with our feelings or emotional dependency on alcohol. You might doubt that you can break up with alcohol for good. Maybe it's the first time you've tried. Perhaps you've tried before and "failed" (affecting your self-confidence).

It's possible that others' opinions may affect you, too. Your intimate drinking circle might advise you negatively about making this change, because they're afraid to lose you as part of their circle, or they may be scared that you're going to change and think differently about them or leave the group altogether. These are realities you may have to deal with as you start living on your terms. As much as you don't want to let your own fears hold you back from growth, you definitely don't want to be held back by *other people's fears.* You can harness the power that comes from uncertainty and transform it into a good energy that propels you toward your goals and desires.

Get to Know Your Fears

Take a moment to think about and write down the specific situations you're afraid of when it comes to reconsidering drinking and breaking up with alcohol. Some examples could be:

- Fear of failure. (*"I can't quit."*)
- Fear of rejection. (*"My friends will cut me out. Nobody will be interested in me or love me if I become sober."*)
- Fear of success. (*"What will my life be like without drinking?"*)
- Fear of boredom. (*"Life without alcohol is life without fun, being a miserable sober."*)
- Fear of missing out on exciting social events. (*"If I'm alcohol free, I won't be included anymore."*)
- Fear of self-sabotage. (*"I thought I would be terrible at this, and I am! I slipped up and had a drink yesterday; all my progress in*

quitting with alcohol is wasted, so I'm going to drink tonight until I pass out.")
- Fear of coping with stress without a drink. (*"I'm under so much pressure, and there's no drinking to counteract it."*)

Use your curiosity to find out what feels uncomfortable and scary about taking this break from alcohol. When you're clear about your fears, where they stem from, and what props them up, you'll be able to *realize what you need to do to overcome them.*

To help you with this, we're going to explain two universal types of fear that everybody is exposed to from time to time: fear of change, and fear of the unknown.

Fear of Change

Fear of change is related to uncertainty about a new reality and our capacity to deal with something unfamiliar that might be beyond our control. You may have this fear if you consistently feel a lack of interest or ability to explore new ideas and situations. As a result, you remain stuck where you are, leading to no change or growth, and eventually, this type of situation harms you.

Other signs of fear of change are when you go to extremes or develop tactics to avoid change; you endure the change but with distress and anxiety; or you use bargaining as an excuse to limit making the change you know is needed. For example, if you know you should break up with alcohol for good, but you keep telling yourself, *"I'll drink during the weekends only,"* or, *"I'll have only two drinks,"* without trying to take any further steps.

Fear of change is universal; everybody experiences it to some degree. It's connected with another widespread fear, the fear of the unknown.

Fear of the Unknown

Fear of the unknown is common to all humans, and it has both positive and negative sides. As a positive, it can be a protective factor, making us cautious and defensive about elements and situations that could represent danger. As a negative, this fear can hold you back, preventing you from experiencing new opportunities or situations that can open your potential and result in growth.

In conclusion, these two basic fears—fear of change and fear of the unknown—will hold you back and put you out of action if you give in to them. You need to *identify and confront these fears*. Sit with the discomfort, face the situation, take the action that makes you feel these fears.

The longer you evade the situation, the harder it becomes to deal with, the bigger the challenge becomes in your mind, and the more your self-confidence is affected. Act with courage, which is not the absence of fear, but *acting while you're scared*, following through on your decision.

If you act with courage, fears can turn into *motivation*. By feeling the fear and taking even one step toward it anyway, you'll experience an increase in your confidence and self-esteem. This will prepare you to face more significant challenges, while enjoying the process and the progress you are making.

Being aware of your fears can act as a *guide*. When you're scared of something, *you're more likely to pay special attention to it,* stay alert, make plans, and look for advice. Pay attention to what causes you to feel fear; be curious about it; respect how you're feeling; follow through and take a step toward the fear anyway.

The Fear Zone and Anger, Bargaining, and Depression

The stages of anger, bargaining, and depression are closely linked to the fear zone, and specifically with the fear of the unknown, when it comes to reconsidering your drinking. In the fear zone, you may be angry, because now that you've gone outside your comfort zone (drinking as much as you wanted), you're aware of how much you're drinking and no longer in denial. You can see clearly the destructive part of your drinking, but you may grapple with wanting to keep drinking anyway, and these realizations may make you feel upset.

Anger is related to fear—fear of being powerless to quit; fear of the destructive consequences if you continue drinking and are unable to stop. Now that you've let yourself confront the destructive reality of alcohol, you may be mad at those around you and blame them for your problems; or you may blame the circumstances surrounding your situation. You may not yet hold your lover (your drink), yourself, or the relationship between you responsible.

Feeling angry is a normal part of the process, and the only way out is through. This process involves acknowledging how alcohol is hurting you and how much is ruined or lost because of drinking.

After anger lessens, another stage you may experience in the fear zone is *bargaining*. The *universal obsession* of people who drink in excess consistently is that one day they'll be able to drink "normally." As part of bargaining, you may ask yourself: What if? *"What if I have only one drink every night? What if I just drink during the weekends? What if I fail and can't make this change?"*

You may miss the good moments with your seductive drink so much that you bargain with yourself in an attempt to have some of those "fun times" again. You may even reach a point where you're willing to forgive and forget all the negative, destructive consequences in exchange for the hope of some more good times. *"I'll drink only two glasses and I'll drink just on Saturdays."* You may fear that you're not up to making the full change you want—whether to reconsider your drinking, take the 21- or 90-day breakup challenge, or be alcohol free. To manage or avoid facing fears—fear of missing out, fear of failure, etc.—you bargain with yourself. You're willing to make some changes that will allow you to continue drinking in some way.

This line of thinking can become a Trojan horse that influences you to relapse with your drinking. If bargaining moves you away from your decision to reconsider your drinking, if it leads you to compromise on what you've agreed to with yourself or excuse yourself from acting on the courage of your convictions, it can be an unsafe coping mechanism. Be aware of the "what ifs" coming up, and keep taking steps toward your goal.

When your anger declines, and you avoid or reject your bargaining ideas, because you realize that they stem from fear and won't help you to change your reality, the depressive stage may begin. In this part of the process, you're aware that you may drink only rarely or perhaps never again, because your drinking is taking more than what you get from it and might cause a serious alcohol use disorder. You know that this lover should go away forever. Your drink will not *be coming back to save you from a bad day at work, or help you deal with friction in your relationship, or keep you relaxed when you're alone at home.*

Acknowledging this reality and the feelings it brings up, *the best idea is to continue moving forward without your drink*, even if you feel there's a void in your life. This is part of the process. It's only a stage, and soon, *things will get better*. Even if it's hard to be in this phase, it will help you to recognize that letting go of your lover and moving on are *part of the healing process*. Pretty soon, the light at the end of the tunnel is going to appear.

Anger, bargaining, and depression can all be related to the fear zone. The best way to deal with the fear of change, the fear of uncertainty, the fear of failure and any other fears that arise is to acknowledge them and continue without giving up. While it's useful to acknowledge fears, we have to make sure we don't pay them too much attention or let them become our main focus. That will allow us to maintain our energy, purpose, and focus on freedom from alcohol.

Specific Fears to Conquer in Reconsidering Your Drinking

We've discussed the two big fears (fear of change, fear of the unknown) you may face in crossing the fear zone. In this section, we let you know some of the specific fears you may face as part of reconsidering your drinking, so that you have the knowledge and confidence to conquer these fears. Chapter 15 provides more detailed suggestions for how to deal with these situations.

- **Fear of losing my day-to-day structure.**
Your drinking may be extremely integrated with your personal and social life. Over the years, drinking may have become a habit with

specific routines. For example: going to a certain store to buy your usual alcoholic drink that you have in a specific place at home, at a certain time, in a special glass; having a select bar where you and your friends typically gather, you know who's coming to hang out, what you're going to order, and so on.

If you're changing a routine, you may experience fear of the unknown: *What happens during this part of the day? What do I do with my time? How will I unwind or socialize? How will I relax or feel comfortable on dates or have fun?* We have to also consider the anticipation of any experiences connected to the routine—the actual drinking; the expectation of fun, camaraderie, or a romantic time, etc.—and their subjective worth.

- **Fear that drinking has already become a severe problem.**

Another fear you may have is that your drinking has become (or is becoming) a serious problem, especially if you already have physical problems related to alcohol (e.g., nausea or shaking when you don't drink), or psychological side effects (e.g., relying on alcohol to deal with problems). If you're already experiencing some physical, mental, or emotional effects related to your drinking, you have two factors to consider: First, quitting alcohol is the best decision to not make the problem worse. Second, you're acting in time to get treatment, heal yourself, and improve your life.

- **Fear that quitting drinking has already become impossible.**

This fear is about already having a physical dependence, and that it will be too difficult to quit. Or that to stop drinking, you'll have to pay for an expensive rehab program. Or that you'll relapse right away. In general, drinking in excess occasionally doesn't imply a physical addiction or alcohol use disorder—even if there is an emotional or psychological dependence, which can be treated and resolved with guidance, therapy, and willpower.

- **Fear that my spouse, partner, or significant other won't connect with me like before.**

This fear can hold you back, so it's important to consider. Chapter 15 contains situation-specific information to help you evaluate and respond to these kinds of circumstances. The resolution of this fear can be unpredictable, as other people are also involved, and the only person you can control is yourself.

As humans, we're always changing, and this is one of our greatest strengths and most remarkable characteristics. Choosing to be alcohol free can lead to changes in your personal relationship with your spouse, partner, or significant other. Routines or activities you've had together that involved drinking will change—whether that's having a glass of wine with dinner, going out for drinks with friends, trying a new bar on the weekend, or having drinks on vacation. This change can affect your interactions, too. Maybe you feel alcohol has been an important part of your communications and bond together, but try to remember that it has certainly also led to, or even created, *difficulties* as well.

It's important to prioritize yourself and your life during this transition. Your relationship with yourself comes first; other relationships come second. You can't keep drinking the same as before just to maintain a relationship or try to make your partner happy.

- **Fear that staying sober is going to be a problem if I'm single and dating.**

You're right that this could be a challenge, and for this reason, many experts recommend not dating until one year after becoming sober. The dating culture in the US is linked closely to alcohol; having a couple of drinks on a first date is almost a must. One of the reasons not to date at the beginning of your new *alcohol-free* life is that the temptation to drink could be too strong, and it could lead you to reconsider drinking again. Besides, you haven't yet formed new alcohol-free habits for dating. So, if this is one of your fears, respect it and give yourself some time to solidify your change and new lifestyle.

- **Fear that I'll face peer pressure regarding drinking.**

Peer pressure about alcohol is a reality in our society, given the normalization of drinking, even of binge drinking when the conditions are "right." When you decide not to drink, you may face *extreme peer pressure to drink again.* You may fear (or experience) being seen as boring, uncool, lame, or an outsider, and this may tempt you to reverse your decision in order to feel accepted again in your social groups.

- **Fear of being invited to bars, parties, or celebrations where drinking is the norm.**

In Chapter 15, we share some suggestions to manage these scenarios, taking into consideration how close you are to the people inviting you and the characteristics of the group regarding drinking.

- **Fear of not looking fun, extroverted, or outgoing.**

We might think that with two or three drinks, we'll look more fun and outgoing, that our shyness will disappear, and we'll look (and feel!) confident socializing with any group. The fear here is about losing the image that you project when drinking, and what that image can connect to (for example, your social capital).

Going outside of your comfort zone is going to expose you to all kinds of fears. Don't underestimate your fears. They can be powerful if you take ownership of them and use them to give you energy, focus, and direction. But if you give your fears control, they'll sabotage your plan, stop your progress, and keep you stuck. If you hold on to your fears to the point that you remain in your comfort zone, you might miss opportunities. Fear will prevent you from living a magnificent life and lower your self-esteem. *Use your fears to work for you*, not against you.

You're going to encounter some roadblocks in this part of the journey, but you're also going to expand into *new aspects of yourself* and have *new insights about yourself and your environment*. You'll realize how strong you are and how great it feels to live life exactly as you want, instead of *reacting to circumstances that make you drink*.

Face your fears one by one, and stay on track with your plan, even if you don't feel great about it. As you keep going, the more confidence you'll have to continue this journey. You'll see that you do have the power and ability on your own, or with others' help (and you can find more tips and resources in Chapter 15), to get through fear. On the other side of the fear zone, you'll find wholeness, growth, freedom, and balance. *The secret is to go through the fear.*

We hope you're proud of yourself for entering and crossing the fear zone. You'll emerge liberated and stronger than ever. Being scared shows you that you're changing, that *you're no longer in that tiny, static, boring comfort zone*. You're healing emotionally, mentally, and physically, and you're gaining confidence to meet your goals.

You are different now! Keep acting on this reality, and, with time, things will get easier and better; your life will open to extraordinary possibilities. *Don't go back to your old comfort zone, to that destructive lover. You have so much to gain in your new and magnificent reality.*

Notes:

CHAPTER 13
EXPLORE THE LEARNING ZONE

"*I started drinking in college, and it was a happy feeling. I come from a closeminded family with a lot of limitations and expectations. Drinking freed me up. I became outgoing and popular. I had a sense of freedom that I could do almost anything, from spending hours at a bar, to singing at midnight in the street, to talking to strangers. My shyness and constraints disappeared, I could express myself in any situation, and I thought I was discovering the 'real me.' I met my husband at a party. We got married and started a comfortable life.*

"*I've changed a lot since then. I used to drink socially, but now I also drink by myself to unwind from the pressures of the day, to avoid thinking about tomorrow, and to relax. I didn't realize that I was developing a bad habit, that many of my daily routines were related to drinking. Still, I was the center of gatherings with friends, girls' weekends, parties, and celebrations, all of which were organized around cocktails. The anticipation of drinking was a happy and comfortable moment, like being in a place you know, where you feel at home.*

"*In reality, nobody knows how much I usually drink. I cross the line almost every night. Long story short: I knew that I had a problem, and*

I decided to quit drinking. I'm enduring this difficult time. I'm hopeful and positive about my life changes and trying to learn what can help me in this process." —Marni

Now that you've identified your fears, you're entering the learning zone. This is where we start exploring our limits, resources, and capabilities to improve future performance, focusing on growth. The goal is to discover and pay attention to the skills you still need to grasp. This means we're trying new things, and mistakes are likely—even encouraged. Failure can be an element of the process. You'll extend your know-how and existing competencies, develop new ones, and *spread your wings*. Through all this, you may feel a bit up in the air and uneasy initially, but it's the way to progress and growth.

When it comes to being free from alcohol, the most significant elements to focus on in the learning zone are (1) understanding why you drink, and (2) expanding your resources and capabilities so you can move forward. This will boost your *self-esteem and confidence*—the motors that keep you going. If your self-esteem and confidence are high, *nothing can stop you*; when they're low, everything looks like an obstacle.

We, as humans, are a work in progress. With learning and development, we become the person we want to be, reaching our full potential and able to accomplish our dreams. When we decide to become alcohol free or to drink in moderation, we focus on what we can gain and open ourselves to a better, thriving future, restoring our health, energy, and vitality. This enables us to have more fulfilling relationships, an improved career, success, and more.

We're choosing to connect with the self and others with deeper authenticity. This is our vision—rather than letting ourselves be trapped in fear that we might *lose* the "fun" we had around drinking, our "enhanced personality," our "exciting routines," or going to particular places to have "good moments" with alcohol. When our life and focus revolved around that old lover, we were losing a lot and stood to lose more and more with time. Because, let's be honest, if our "fun" was dependent on alcohol, how real was that experience, and how long could it last? It's astonishing how, when we love something or someone, we pay little or no attention to their faults.

Now that you've embraced this adventure fully, you're learning to replace that seductive but conflictual lover. There are *other beverages* you can choose from; there are many ways to *manage social situations* involving alcohol; there are other *habits and routines* you can adopt. By discovering and learning the new steps that are required, you're entering a new life in which you'll gain and not lose, as before. *You're going to live on your own terms; alcohol won't be the deciding factor for you anymore.*

The more we learn, take action, and move forward in a new stage, the more freedom and flexibility we experience. It won't be like in the past, when we were stuck with the drink, with *nothing more than what alcohol gave us at that moment*, which on its own already brought harmful, problematic factors into our life.

Learning new steps and taking action will be the key to our progress during this stage, because it will open us to realities that may include exciting and valuable tools. Through this process, we'll experience freedom from our old habits and, at the same time, a sense of grounding and inclusion into new opportunities and routines, a feeling of liberation from that poison, which is no longer a component of our life.

It's possible that in the past, when you were in your comfort zone with the drink, rather than learning, *you were repeating*, again and again, the same scenarios, routines, conversations, and problems. Now that you've decided to leave that superficially cozy reality, there are two factors that might bring up difficult emotions, such as grief, anger, or blame: (1) The ideas that you had regarding alcohol as happy and fun, and (2) that you were well on the way toward developing an addiction without realizing it. It may be hard to get over these, because the person you have to accept when you wake up in the morning is *you*. But see if, alongside the awareness, you can bring a sense of understanding and self-compassion toward yourself for:

- Creating a false idealization of alcohol, thinking that it brings happiness (when in reality, this lover brings problems).
- Not thinking alcohol was so addictive (now you know that human willpower is limited when facing something that creates cravings and dependence).

Now that you have more information and tools, you can do more to help yourself. We want you to build a mindset that inspires you to be centered, courageous, open-minded, and full of clarity. *Rather than letting drinking drag you down; you can be the one rising above, conquering obstacles and reaching new horizons.* You'll get to your happy place when you're choosing the life you want—*free, magnificent, yours!*

What You Need to Discover and Learn When Becoming Alcohol Free

You'll be more successful in your journey to a happy alcohol-free life if your expectations are based on reality. The rest of this chapter will cover the factors you might experience and need to learn and work on to get through this zone with greater ease.

Chapter 13: Explore the Learning Zone

What You Can Expect to Encounter

1. People might think that you've quit drinking because you previously had a problem with alcohol.

This is a frequent assumption: that you've stopped drinking because you were an alcoholic or close. If other people's opinions are important to you (as is true for many of us), you may want to have a solid reason.

Of course, you don't *have to* give any explanation. You might feel it's no one else's business what you put in your body. You can also avoid the subject altogether, if you want, or until you know for sure what your relationship with alcohol will be or what you're comfortable with explaining. It's your life, and you've decided to live on your terms. *Focus on you and your needs, not on others' opinions.*

2. People might be uncomfortable and upset with your not drinking.

Many people are going to be upset and uncomfortable with your decision. They may react in unexpected ways, from surprise and suspicion, to incredulity, cynicism, and more. Common themes in others' responses are:

- *You're not an alcoholic, so why don't you drink with us, if you don't have a problem?*
- *You're missing out on all the fun we usually have.*
- *If you don't drink, you're not "one of us."*
- *We don't want you in our group anymore, because not only are you not fun but also you'll be judging us for how much we drink.*
- *It's challenging to have you as part of the group; you're different from us, and we don't feel we can connect with you in the same ways.*

The majority of the messages we receive from society, our community, peers, and sometimes even our family imply that drinking is good and helps us to relax, have fun, celebrate, and enhance our personality. The only "valid" reasons that justify being alcohol free is if you are or were an alcoholic, are unable to control your drinking, or have a health issue, which means that *you're not doing okay and you have no choice.*

You can tell people that you want to live your life at its best without the numbing effects of alcohol, and that you can have wonderful moments without the booze. It's okay to show how happy you feel making this decision and how proud of yourself you are because of it.

If people around you judge or exclude you, this can be tough in the moment, but *try not to take it personally.* It's normal that not everyone will want to hang out with us, nor us with them, and that's okay; it happens to us all. Keep doing what you've decided in an unapologetic way; it's your life, and you have the right to decide what's best for you.

3. You may feel uncomfortable around heavy drinkers.

Once you've broken up with that lover, alcohol, being around other drinkers, especially heavy drinkers, can feel like being in another reality. You might feel distant and different from drinkers. You may feel sorry for their behaviors, traditions, and rituals, knowing that sooner or later, they will experience problems and negative consequences. Also, you may be sorry for the years you were that way, too. You may be wondering why it took you so long to make the decision to quit. But stay present—*you did it!*

Additionally, you may feel uncomfortable if some consequences of alcohol use occur in your presence (e.g., vomiting, falling down, talking nonsense), or if you hear about events or experiences relating to alcohol use that you may have thought were fun but now perceive as repetitive, gross, rude, or vulgar. You don't want to act like that anymore or have those same problems and consequences. You may feel lonely and alienated, like *the only one who can see the truth about alcohol*. It's important to keep reminding yourself that you've made the best decision.

4. Sobriety doesn't fix everything.

The truth is that, of course, you'll continue to experience ups and downs and face problems after you quit drinking, because you're human and living life. But here's the thing: Without alcohol dominating your life, you'll have greater clarity in your thoughts and emotions, which will allow you *to more easily return to your center and wholeness as many times as you need to.*

Being in the learning zone may be a powerful time to resolve any issues triggered by your past drinking; for example: mending relationships, spending more time with your kids and family, focusing on your job or career, getting healthier, sleeping better, losing weight, and finding new interests and positive people to spend your time with.

Without alcohol-induced brain fog, confusion, misperceptions, misunderstandings, or mix-ups, more options will be available to you. You'll enjoy more time without the invalidating or constrictive consequences of hangovers. You'll have more freedom in all aspects of your life. These benefits will *better prepare you to evaluate situations, find solutions, let things go more easily, set and manage your boundaries, or even disregard a matter* if you choose to.

5. Alcohol-free dating is challenging.

Yes, it is! For that reason, as we've recommended, it's totally okay to take a break from dating or to go slowly, given the characteristics of the dating culture in the US and many other places. In the US, dating and drinking go hand to hand; most dates happen in bars or restaurants where drinking is almost (or can feel like) a must.

Connecting with someone else without the effects of alcohol can be wonderful. Your senses are working without impairment; you may be more present and better able to tell if there's real attraction, affinity, and similar interests; if your personalities and lifestyles are compatible; if there's potential for a long-term relationship.

What You Can Expect to Discover

1. The first steps are the most difficult.

At the beginning of your breakup with alcohol, you may feel that you won't be happy again, that life will be boring, that you'll become introverted and lonely—or other variations of limiting beliefs (refer back to the list you made for yourself in Chapter 10).

Part of the challenge in the learning zone is that you have *to break with some old habits and learn something new*. Humans are creatures of habit, and when a habit is formed, all the behaviors related to it become a necessity.

Say, for instance, that we're in the habit of drinking coffee first thing in the morning. Having coffee as soon as we wake up is something we need; we can't start our day without a cup of joe. What do we do if we decide not to drink coffee again? First, maybe we freak out. Then we look for alternative morning drinks, such as tea, smoothies, or juices. We learn what's available and how to prepare it. We try different things and see what we like best. With time, we can find a good coffee replacement that makes us happy. We have to point out that if there's a caffeine addiction, there will be withdrawal symptoms that will go away with time.

The same happens with the booze. We've gotten into the habit of drinking, so we "need" our wine, beer, or cocktail at certain times or in specific situations. This habit was developed based on *learned behavior and has become unconscious.*

Now we must *release the habit in a conscious way,* which is going to require effort from you (see Chapter 15 for our suggestions). All the work you've been doing and the steps you've taken so far are to empower you to break free from the habit of drinking. This is a huge step that opens the possibility of learning new positive habits that will unlock new frontiers.

When I, Pilar, decided to quit drinking, I started thinking about what could replace my favorite white wine. I tried several beverages, and finally, I settled on kombucha. This is now my favorite drink at the end of my day, when I get together with friends, or attend gatherings and parties. I started by buying kombucha and having fun with trying new flavors. Then I bought a book and learned how to brew kombucha at home. Right now I like kombucha way more than a good dry white wine. The only problem is that some restaurants and bars don't have kombucha (yet), so when going out, I make a point to pick places that offer it.

You can see that Pilar changed her focus. Instead of stopping at the point of missing her wine, she tried other beverages and found a new drink that she liked and kept exploring. As a result, she now has a new hobby of brewing kombucha at home and dedicates time to this skill, rather than focusing on what is gone from her life. *Replace a loser with a winner.*

2. There are other alcohol-free people.

Sobriety is trending in our society, and there are more and more fascinating people who are following this path. Look around you, go online, walk, hike, backpack, jog, run, or attend a workout or a yoga class, and you'll find numerous people of all ages who are taking your exact route and with whom you can share your experiences. Being alcohol free will open the door to meeting people and making new friends. In time, you'll probably question how you ever lived without them. You'll be surprised by all the wonderful people who will enter your life *because* you decided to stop drinking. And guess what? People living an alcohol-free lifestyle *are not* "miserable sobers." They have happy and fulfilling lives; they're generally successful at what they do; they have interesting hobbies; they're healthy. From our professional experience, *not a single one regrets the decision not to drink.*

3. Sharing your thoughts and feelings with others will help you in the journey.

Becoming alcohol free is a deeply personal decision. Sometimes, the reasons for this change are apparent, while others might be subconscious. Sharing your thoughts and feelings with others, both close friends or new people you meet, might help you to clarify many elements of your reality and see how you relate to others' experiences as well.

During these conversations, you might discuss why you made the decision, whether it's a temporary break or a permanent one; your worries about the before and after; your knowledge about addiction; new routines; other beverages; and how you see your future without alcohol. Listening to yourself talk about the positives of an alcohol-free life—and the opposite, the negatives of continuing to drink—*subconsciously strengthens your commitment to the decision.*

A critical component of sharing with others is that you become conscious of essential parts of yourself. You'll realize that you know more about yourself than you'd thought and that the information you have is reinforced through sharing. This awareness is crucial for your self-esteem and self-confidence, awakening and strengthening these elements within you, which is vital to dealing with present and future challenges.

Conversations and interactions with others will help you to build and reinforce your new identity and develop specific new values and routines for your life. *You'll bolster yourself and provide inspiration for others.*

4. Your alcohol-free life is your responsibility.

Being sober can be a limitation or a liberation. It's *your choice*. You decide. It's in your hands. We encourage you to see your sobriety as *personal growth*. It's also something that doesn't start and end with you alone. You can inspire others to reconsider their drinking and be alcohol free, always appreciating how much life is improving when not under the influence of that destructive habit.

What You Need to Learn

1. What's a good replacement drink for you?

There are nonalcoholic beer, wine, and cocktail selections at almost any liquor store, with many options. Some people also enjoy other beverages like sparkling water, kombucha, juices, and mocktails.

2. How do you recreate your day-to-day structure?

For many of us, our personal and social life was structured around drinking. *This structure goes down like a house of cards once we decide to quit alcohol.* This is just one indication that the design was *unreliable and unstable*, much like our reality when we're under the influence of alcohol.

In this case, the collapse is a good thing—a clean sweep. Why? Because *you've chosen this journey* with the purpose of reconstructing your life *using something better, something real and solid*—building a new path for yourself, and consequently a much better present and future.

Anyway—and *pay attention to this*—your past structure was likely to fall apart and collapse at *any* moment. It was a matter of time. Because you have orchestrated this breakdown intentionally with your positive change, you can use it to your advantage, as a time to create growth and new resources and tap into existing strengths while building your new life structure and identity.

Be aware that you may be or become a different person without your drinking. As a result, *you'll head down a different path in your life, with new routines, people, and activities.* If you try to go on the same as before, you'll feel that something is missing and experience the same desires and cravings as in the past. At that point there's a chance that, if you don't evolve, you may start drinking again, and your drink may fully control your life once more.

3. How do you change or reconstruct your intimate/personal relationship?

"My husband and I have been married for twenty years, and we couldn't have children. What we missed with not being able to raise kids, we replaced with an exciting connection between us. We lived in a small apartment for years while we were starting our careers. Gradually, we improved our lives until we were able to buy a beautiful house with a wonderful swimming pool. We were grateful for all of that. We started ending our day with a drink in our backyard. This was our own happy hour, when we shared our day, what we were going to eat for dinner, our expectations for tomorrow, and any reciprocal comments or advice. But through the years, two drinks were not enough. If there was something special (good or bad), we continued with one or two more drinks. Now I want to quit, because I know this isn't good for me in the long run. But since the happy hours and drinks are such an important part of our time to connect in our relationship, how can I deal with this with my husband? I'm afraid he'll be upset and unsupportive of the idea of being alcohol free." —Desiree

If drinking is something that you do with your partner and both of you want to quit, obviously you should find another activity or routine to do together that can replace the drink, perhaps something you do in a different environment. This is a situation that requires deep conversations to reach a point where you both agree and feel excited about the change.

If the two of you are in different stages—if only one of you wants to take a break from alcohol—you'll have to give special attention to the reasons and consequences, because it's possible that the entire dynamic of your relationship might change.

Consider that alcohol can have a harmful effect on relationships in the following situations:

- If there's a *lack of honesty* about the drinking. Especially if one of you is lying or hiding alcohol intake from the other, it's a sign that alcohol is having a negative effect on each of you *and* on the relationship. This scenario creates an "affair" situation—alcohol becomes the "other person" with whom a partner in the relationship is cheating. With time, hiding the alcohol becomes normal, and relationships disintegrate under this dynamic.
- If drinking *provokes or increases conflict*. Under the influence of alcohol, we're more impulsive, and the possibility of self-control decreases. How many conflicts and fights can be avoided if alcohol is removed from the picture?
- If drinking is a *central part* of the relationship. Like any other important factor in a couple's life, drinking should be kept in check by both members of the pair, who should be each other's safeguard and boundary, taking into account that alcohol is addictive.

4. How to be an alcohol-free single and deal with dating?

We know that *dating without drinks is possible.* In fact, it could set you up for better connections, because you have all of your senses intact, and alcohol is not altering your personality. Dating without alcohol can be the start of a healthy long-term relationship.

The first thing to consider is whether *you're ready* for a new relationship. If you've decided to be alcohol free, you're experiencing many changes in your life and are in a period of transition and adjustment, learning and unlearning about yourself.

Keep in mind that some people won't be a fit with your new lifestyle; some might not agree with or understand the change and growth you're experiencing. You might feel lonely or bored once you've ended your relationship with alcohol and think that a romantic relationship is the way to overcome those feelings. Be aware that this *is not a right reason* to look for love. Our recommendations are in Chapter 15.

5. How do I deal with peer pressure?

"For years I've had a wonderful circle of friends. We're all from different backgrounds and have different ages and personalities, but we've supported and encouraged each other. I've been through many difficult situations, starting with my mother's death, and most recently, a divorce. During those times, I relied on wine and my girlfriends (who all drink) to get through the stress and pain. But as time passed, and after some minor incidents, I realized I wanted to take a new approach.

"When I talked with one of my best friends, Diane, about taking a break from drinking, she reacted in a way that made things even worse. It was like she didn't want me to change, and not having her support made me doubt my ability to succeed. She brought up the topic within the group, and everybody was on her side. I felt that they didn't approve of the new me, and that made me rethink my goal of maintaining my sobriety.

"Now I know why Diane was not supporting me in my decision to become alcohol free: She was pulling me into the past to keep me in her life. She was afraid that I would drift away if I changed and stayed sober. Her fear of losing me was guiding her actions, but how did her friendship become a selfish attachment? Only because I wanted to quit drinking and make my life better." —Silvia

Our friends and colleagues might still be going along with the societal "normalization" of drinking and embrace drinking as a norm, which leads them to see you as missing out, an outsider, or not trustworthy. You can't be *"one of us"* if you're sober, and they will only accept your alcohol-free status if you are or were an active alcoholic or have a credible excuse. There can be a lot of peer pressure in this space.

We have some concrete advice in Chapter 15 for facing peer pressure. Our hope for you is that you live your alcohol-free life with authenticity and use this change as an opportunity to grow and live in a better way. Consequently, you *won't* have to worry about peer pressures. You'll be on another level, not held down by a *"poor me" mindset (attitude)*, scared of the social backlash. You'll live with *the high of a stunning mindset*—able to make changes in your life and full of confidence and happiness with the direction you're taking.

6. How can I be part of parties and celebrations without drinking?

Same as before: *Go to the party and have fun!* You don't need everybody's support and approval for what you are or aren't drinking. Chances are, you're going to enjoy parties and celebrations even more, as you're not under the disinhibition provoked by alcohol, and tomorrow, when you wake up, you won't be worrying about whether alcohol affected what you said or did. You're going to awake fresh and happy, feeling confident that you acted with authenticity and delighted, remembering the great party you attended.

Notes:

CHAPTER 14
ENTER THE GROWTH ZONE

As our personal development continues, we enter the growth zone, where our intentions and actions are guided by clear goals directed to our growth. Our life starts gaining more clarity and meaning as our vision develops along with new capacities and talents. Fears evaporate as we learn how to deal with our new reality. We see stumbles and setbacks as opportunities to learn. This increases our resilience and self-confidence to look forward, and our motivations and mindset expand positively with new aspirations. These are some of the indications that we're in the growth zone.

"I notice that when I face situations without alcohol that used to feel uncomfortable or like I couldn't do it—for example, going on a date or an evening out with friends, or relaxing at the end of the day—they're not nearly as bad or difficult as I had feared. So, I realized that I'm not in the fear zone anymore. Sure, I've needed to learn some things, but it hasn't been too difficult.

"For me, the main thing was to change the way I felt about alcohol. One day, I was looking for something online, and I saw a questionnaire about crossing the line with drinking. Until then, I'd thought of myself

as a 'social drinker.' That questionnaire showed me that I was in a dangerous situation—drinking in excess too often and on the way to becoming addicted.

"How did I change the way I felt about alcohol? My whole adult life, I'd believed that alcohol helped me in my personal and social life. When I was with others, it made me more fun and charming. When I was by myself, it helped me relax and unwind from the tensions of the day. While I was drinking, I had some fun moments with my partner, but it also led to some arguments. In general, my mindset about alcohol was that I was gaining something with it—good moments, relationships, acceptance—until I realized that I was losing a lot. Not seeing that I was crossing a line was part of my denial.

"I remember that I'd had some moments of clarity—when I'd put empty bottles in the trash, or in the middle of the day out of the blue, or when I awoke at 4:00 a.m. with insomnia and a headache. I sobered up because of one of those moments the day after I decided to take that questionnaire. Before that, I'd said to myself, 'I'll drink less next week, I'll take a break next month,' or 'I'm not that bad. Give up drinking? Give up all the awesome things and social life that comes with it? Never!' It had become part of my identity, my environment, my schedule.

"When I started to realize that I could have all these things, and in even better ways, without drinking, I began to change, and I thought I could quit. I have changed since then. I'm not the same person anymore. Enough was enough. I decided to change my life for the better." —Matilda

By now, you have decided to take a break from alcohol. It was a difficult decision, but after the initial shock, you could see beyond your denial to how destructive alcohol is. You could control your anger, and you got past the temptation to use bargaining to avoid change. Then, the difficult part came when you felt depressed, because you were no longer drinking. But you forged ahead, and you started accepting that your lover, your drink, would not return to you anymore, and that the destruction this relationship caused was behind you.

Through this journey, you've faced your fears, you've learned what you needed to know. You didn't get stuck in limiting beliefs, and with your positive mindset, you've rapidly made new discoveries. Since you know that you're not a victim, you don't blame anybody or anything else; you recognize that what happened before was your responsibility. You also see that the necessary changes and bright future you desire are within your power and reach.

Now you're here, in the growth zone, with clear thoughts, conscious of your emotions and feelings, and action-oriented regarding your intentions and goals. You've decided to reconsider your drinking or to quit altogether, and you feel *free*, with more physical and mental energy. You're at the stage where you can develop your full potential.

First things first: You've made an *excellent choice*! In all our years of combined professional practice—psychological and medical private practice, coaching, and running a program for psychiatric rehabilitation—*not one of our patients or clients has regretted making this change.*

Second, the key to success is *to keep things simple*. Stick to the essentials. Identify the key points or circumstances to prioritize. Do this with as much *humility and self-compassion* as possible.

Plan Ahead to Set Yourself up for Success

In general, *doing anything new for the first time is usually the most difficult time*. Identify your weak points and the situations in your life that can make you vulnerable to drinking again. Consider the highs and lows when you would have previously liked to drink and when you're tempted to do so now. We believe in *anticipating difficult situations*, which requires thinking in advance and preparing yourself with the right internal and external tools.

For example, during your first alcohol-free year, there will be holidays and celebrations that traditionally include alcohol, such as New Year's Eve, when you might be tempted to drink. Have a plan in advance. Try celebrating with a spectacular brunch on January 1 instead of getting wasted on December 31 and having a painful hangover to start the new year.

To identify these types of key points in your life, you must think about past experiences when it was "essential" for you to have a drink or you didn't feel you could say no. We're all different, so this identification is *very personal*.

Try it...

Think of three hypothetical times or situations in which you would like a drink. Here are some examples:
- During happy events.
- During unhappy times.
- To forget problems or worries.
- For confidence.
- To relax and unwind.
- For friendship.
- To feel sophisticated.
- To get through heartbreak.
- On dates.
- With your partner, to connect and share a moment together.

- When you're cooking.
- To stop your mind racing.
- To feel better.
- When you're at home.
- During lonely times when your drink is your lover.
- During weekends or special days.
- On vacation.
- During celebrations.
- During holidays.

In the following case, drinking was linked to a heartbreak:

"I started dating James two years ago. We met through mutual friends, and slowly we realized our companionship was turning into something else. We had so much in common; we could talk about anything, and we frequently had good laughs because of a similar sense of humor. For the first time after my divorce, I was interested in somebody. At the same time, I felt scared of what the future might hold for this relationship. Was it going to continue? Would it become a partnership? Pretty soon, I had an answer to my internal questions. James's replies to my texts came later and became shorter. When I asked why, he said he was busy. This continued until the point that he didn't answer anymore. I was desperate and had one question: What did I do wrong?

"At that time, my coping mechanism was drinking by myself or with friends. I wanted to understand what happened, but James just vanished without giving me closure. If we had talked, maybe it would have been easier to move on, but as it was, the situation felt so negative and incomprehensible for me. I was using drinking to replace him, but I knew this wasn't a healthy or long-term solution. Already, I was paying for it the next day with hangovers, headaches, and low energy." —Katie

If you know what your high and low points are, you can plan for how to deal with them. Being prepared will give you the necessary confidence to face these events or circumstances, and your efforts will be rewarded with heightened self-esteem and confidence *("I did it!")*.

Again, remember that that the first time (or few first times) we tackle something related to our vulnerabilities is usually the most difficult. But don't let that discourage or stop you. Instead, let the fact that you can spot the challenge and create and enact a plan give you confidence that you're acting according to your ideals and goals.

As part of this plan, you will need to:
- Stop any self-sabotaging thoughts or behaviors.
- Consolidate your decisions with action.
- Promote personal growth aligned with your purposes.

Let's return to Katie:

"I'm still working on forgiving, forgetting, and moving on from this painful situation. But I'm going to stop turning to alcohol. I'll ask James if we can talk about our relationship and his reasons for ending communications and leaving. But no matter what he says, my actions and self-care are not based on him or whether he agrees to talk. I can keep going.

"I'll think, or look for consultation, about the elements that are under my control and those that aren't. I'll give myself time to express gratitude for the good moments I had, for the growth that the experience gave me, and accept the reality that the relationship has come to a close. I'll seek to heal my wounds, pull my life together, and move on, understanding that alcohol would just numb me and delay this process."

In conclusion, and turning the focus back to you: What are the *high points* that would have previously caused you to reach for a drink?

What are the *low points* that could make you sabotage your progress? What *internal and external resources* can you use to choose a path and coping mechanisms or actions other than drinking? Make a plan for each of these situations, as Katie did.

Notes:

CHAPTER 15

GUIDANCE FOR SPECIFIC CHALLENGES AND SITUATIONS

As you continue your journey of becoming alcohol free, the information, tools, and resources in this chapter will help you to increase your confidence, consolidate your progress, and plan ahead. Just as "chance favors the prepared," *never underestimate the power of being ready to confront difficult situations.* Breaking up with alcohol can be a particularly arduous decision because it requires consideration and care of both internal and external factors. We're going to outline some of the specific situations and challenges that you may face around socializing and solitude when you reconsider your drinking, and we'll share ideas that will help you prepare for success.

We discuss how to deal with everyday personal and social life issues, social connections and special events that traditionally involve alcohol, like dating, vacations, holidays, and celebrations. We include occasion-specific tips for how you can be comfortable in your own skin while not drinking, especially if you were convinced previously that alcohol is what made you feel fun and outgoing. We share suggestions for how to get through difficult times without alcohol, especially if a drink is what you used to go to for comfort, and how to deal with the times when you used to drink by yourself.

Release the Habit of Drinking

We understand that drinking is a *habit* we've gotten into, "needing" our wine, beer, or cocktail at certain times or for specific occasions, no matter what. It's essential to *release that habit in a conscious way.*

As we challenged you in Chapter 8, the best way to make this tangible change is to take at least twenty-one consecutive days without drinking. If you miss a day, that's okay; just start the twenty-one days over again, and keep going until you've had a full twenty-one consecutive days without alcohol. Ideally, we recommend at least three months of not drinking to consolidate your practice of being alcohol free, and to see a lifestyle change, per the "21/90 rule" (see Chapter 8). Look at this time as a chance to practice a discipline that gives you freedom, real connection with yourself and others, and better health. As you persevere, you'll find that you no longer suffer the feelings of dependency and urges that kept you tied to that destructive lover.

To break free, consolidate this change, and move forward, you need *to create new routines and engage in new activities* to replace the drinking-focused habits you had before. For example:
- If you used to drink in the evenings at home after work, what routines and activities will replace those hours at home? You might use the time to work out, go for a walk, attend a yoga or meditation class, try a new hobby, declutter your home, learn a new language, take an art class, get some career education or training, volunteer, spend time outdoors, play with your kids, read a book, or some

- combination of these or other activities. Be focused and specific.
- If you used to go to happy hours, restaurants, or bars, where will you go and what will you do instead during those times? Could you go on a hike, take a class, meet a friend, go shopping or do another activity using the money you've saved by not drinking alcohol?
- If you used to favor particular alcoholic beverages, what non-alcoholic drinks could you enjoy instead?

It will be hard to make a lasting change if you quit just alcohol but try to keep everything else the same. The key to success is to replace old habits and routines with new ones.

There are two main components to creating your long-term alcohol-free identity:

(1) Replace your old habits and routines around drinking with new activities.

(2) Replace your drink with nonalcoholic drinks you enjoy.

You may try something new and find that you don't enjoy it or it's not the right fit. *That's okay.* Keep testing new things until you find something you like to replace the routines and hours centered on drinking. Building new, healthier habits is an important step to free us from the habit of drinking and to open new possibilities. Establishing *new positive habits* will *unlock new frontiers.*

Create New Habits and Routines

Drinking can be so integrated into both regular and special days that quitting often requires and creates change in our day-to-day experience. You'll need to find new routines to replace old ones—for instance, going for a walk instead of going to a bar, getting up early to do something instead of staying up late drinking.

We must *build a new structure* for ourselves that doesn't revolve around drinking. You don't have to come up with a plan all at once, but now is the beginning of a process in which we encourage you *to think about and connect with ideas that excite and motivate you*. Use these ideas to create plans and, slowly but surely, start to fill the empty space.

Be curious about what's going on inside and around you and create new inner connections in your relationship to yourself until you start to find a silver lining. Following are some tips to help you with this:

- *Find a role model.* Who has made this change in an effective way? Can you contact that person and ask for guidance? Follow the advice of others who have walked this journey; imitate; follow the process.
- *Know your triggers.* When do you really feel you need a drink? Is it connected to times of the day, days of the week, stressful situations, being with certain people, traditions, celebrations, holidays, etc.? When you have clarity about what sets off your desire to drink, strategize, and be prepared to manage and respond to those situations in the best way you can—always from the perspective of *what you stand to gain*; never operating from a place of loss.
- *Do things that bring you joy.* Find new activities, places, experiences, and people that make you happy. Learn to enjoy your own company. Schedule fun. Connect often with these resources.
- *Be confident and optimistic.* Without alcohol, your future is much brighter, healthier, and happier! You're setting yourself up for a more fulfilling life.
- *Find projects that interest you.* Hobbies are great during this stage. What's something you've always wanted to try that you can do

Chapter 15: Guidance for Specific Challenges and Situations

for the first time? Or maybe there's something you used to enjoy that you can start up again? Find things that help you to get into a state of flow.[45]

- *Enjoy challenges.* They help you grow and expand.
- *Be grateful.* You have this opportunity to turn your life around. *It's a gift.* In a few months, and certainly a year from now and into the future, you'll be so proud of yourself for making this decision.

We want to share with you three success stories from our clients to provide some examples you can use to plan new routines and activities to replace your drinking habits. Believe that you must do this to improve your life. It's challenging but definitely possible and within your reach.

Brooke struggled during the first week she decided to go alcohol free. For the past ten years, her evening routine involved putting her children to bed and having a few drinks right after, from 8:30 p.m. until her own bedtime of 11:30 p.m. Without her usual evening drinks, she felt empty, anxious, and bored. She decided that she was going to get more sleep every night, and moved her bedtime up to 10:00 p.m. This also meant that the hours she previously used to spend drinking were reduced to one-and-a-half hours only. She put other activities into her evening routine: decluttering her home for thirty minutes, doing an online yoga class, or taking a hot bath.

She persevered through the discomfort of the first week, and around day ten, she realized that she was feeling rested and relaxed, and she was getting her house in order! After a month she felt like never before,

---

45. A flow state can arise when we're immersed in an experience that takes our effort and skill. We're totally present in the activity, and our attention is so fully absorbed that we may even lose track of time.

sleeping for eight hours per night consistently. She used the money saved from not buying her usual wine to purchase new décor items, so her home space was also improving. She felt like this was the most powerful reset of her life. She was healthier and had more energy. She even started working out again after years of sedentary life.

Brooke improved her health, sleep, physical state, and home environment by not drinking alcohol anymore and replacing that habit with new, healthy routines. *If you used to drink at home like Brooke, can you create new habits and routines as she did?*

Giselle loved having drinks while cooking dinner every evening for her and her husband. Soon after deciding to stop drinking, she convinced her husband Brad to take a break from drinking with her and to work out together with the goal of losing five pounds in three weeks. Brad wanted to support her, so he embraced the plan.

They decided that they were going to try an hour-long workout at their local gym to fill the time they previously spent cooking and having drinks together. They added fifteen minutes of walking, and sometimes wrapped up their exercise at the gym hot tub. After that, they went home and had a healthy meal while watching TV. They went to bed right after, earlier than normal.

The gym routine was not easy, but they stuck to it, and after the second week they felt great. The extra sleep, healthy food, workouts, walks, and hot tub time increased their well-being. In three weeks, they surpassed their weight loss goal! They decided to continue their evening workout and hot tub routine several days per week. The money they saved from not buying alcohol helped them to book a Caribbean vacation that had been on their bucket list for a long time. Giselle and Brad experienced such positive changes that they decided to stay alcohol-free forever. *Can you put the money you save by not drinking alcohol toward something else you want? Do you have a partner or buddy you can enlist to make the changes with you, as Giselle did?*

Carla, a single woman, used to drink heavily during weekends, going out on Fridays and hanging with friends on Saturdays and Sundays, drinking for long hours and starting the workweek on Mondays with no energy.

To break her drinking habit, she decided to hike on the weekends and joined a local club that organized regular group hikes. It was hard at the beginning, as she had no prior experience, but she got stronger with time, and added a yoga class every Friday night. She took a break from her usual drinking social circle, stating that she wanted to get healthier. Secretly, hiking was something she'd actually wanted to do for a long time, but never had time or money for before because of her social life and how much she was drinking.

Carla put the money she saved by not buying alcohol toward the gear she needed for hiking and camping. She started traveling to state and national parks and fell in love with her new lifestyle. She met new people and struck up solid friendships with a new group that are now her tribe. She also met the love of her life, a guy who was a long-time hiker. They decided to be outdoors as much as possible, move in together, and stay alcohol free. *How can you redirect the energy and time you used to spend on drinking toward something else you want to do for your health, as Carla did?*

If your situation is similar to Brooke, Giselle, or Carla's stories, *can you relate to the changes they made and how they decided to incorporate new routines and activities to support their new lifestyle?*

Choose a Replacement Beverage

Think about what beverage will replace your favorite alcoholic drink, be it wine, beer, spirits, or cocktails. *This is crucial. You need a good replacement drink that contains no alcohol. Period.*

You can look for healthy drinks like kombucha, fresh juices, and creative mocktails; or conventional drinks such as iced tea, sparkling water, soda with lemon or lime, cranberry juice, apple juice, or water with a splash of pineapple. Going further, you can choose a virgin cocktail or a nonalcoholic beer or wine. Perhaps you'll have a few nonalcoholic go-tos. Find what you like, and have that beverage available at home or to bring with you to events so that you'll always have your new drink available.

Rewire Expectations

Expectations can be powerful and create both positive and negative consequences. Good expectations lead us to move forward and make progress in life. Negative or unrealistic expectations can keep us *stuck in a place that's unhealthy for us*. Expectations about alcohol (for example, societal pressure to drink, the normalization of alcohol, "alcohol equals good times") can be both powerful and negative in that they prevent *us from making a change to reconsider and quit drinking*. Alcohol keeps us stuck.

Before, you may have expected a lot from your drink, and it seemed that alcohol could deliver what you wanted, such as:

- A relaxed moment.
- Coziness.
- A fun evening.
- A less lonely time at home.
- A fun get-together.

Chapter 15: Guidance for Specific Challenges and Situations

- A way to end your long day.
- A way to stop your mind.

You recognize now that your expectations for alcohol *didn't include the feelings of the day after*, such as hangovers, regrets, shame, and negative consequences; or the impacts to our health that result from drinking. But when you thought you were getting what you wanted from alcohol, your expectations prompted you to drink more and more without much acknowledgment of the negative consequences.

You also understand that those pleasant effects can't necessarily be attributed to alcohol and that you can experience them through other means. However, your mind and body may still connect those positive results to alcohol. Even though you're reconsidering your drinking and making changes to drink moderately or be alcohol free, this is a new venture. It takes time to rewire your expectations so that you *connect those pleasant feelings to other sources.*

What will you do when you feel bored, lonely, or stressed out? What will you do when you go to a get-together, and everybody drinks? What's your new plan? We need to *both exclude alcohol* and *create a new set of expectations, activities, and routines that we connect to an alcohol-free lifestyle and the positive effects we desire.* You can use this new mental map to replace the old expectations (and don't forget to include the negative consequences) of what you used to get when crossing the line with alcohol.

Rewiring your expectations and how you meet them is *key* to not going back to alcohol again and potentially drinking more than before. It isn't easy, but you'll become more practiced and comfortable with time, until you realize how much is out there and how great it feels when you're not under the influence.

As you continue this program, challenge all your expectations of your drinking, being open to thinking critically about how you feel at each moment you decide not to drink. Look for the old patterns and expectations and question whether they are true. Acknowledge the negative consequences of alcohol that have a place in your old expectations, and factor this into your decision-making. Work on building *a new set of expectations and activities* that you connect to being alcohol free, knowing that everyone who has decided to be alcohol free has gone through the same situation.

Manage Social Pressures

How to Respond to Peer Pressure

Family and Close Friends: You might share your decision with close family and friends and ask for their support. Your alcohol-free choice is nothing to be ashamed of. For anyone you're interested in keeping in your life, don't hide your sobriety or make excuses! Be yourself, *sincere and proud* about who you are and your decision. Ideally, you'll get acceptance from your friends so that they relate to and/or support your new alcohol-free identity and lifestyle.

At the same time, we know that people who choose to be alcohol free typically face peer pressure, including from their close circle. Boundaries are important. If interacting with your friends who drink feels too intense or negative, you could take a break from hanging out with them until you feel more established on your alcohol-free journey. Another possibility is to look for new friends who may be more aligned with and supportive of your new reality and future lifestyle.

Acquaintances: With people who are your acquaintances, colleagues, or coworkers, you may or may not choose to disclose your decision, or you might give some other reason for not drinking (for example: needing to get up early tomorrow, "not feeling it tonight," responding with humor).

We don't usually place as much stock in opinions from people we don't know well. So, if peer pressure comes from people you *aren't* close to, proceed as with other aspects of your life. Communicate *only* what you want to share. Don't react to their shock, misinterpretation, or confusion about being alcohol free. Don't create a storyline of being either a victim or a victor; rather, see yourself as someone with the *right and responsibility to make your own decisions* and to live as you want.

Groups: If group dynamics are such that drinking isn't "required," it's fine to say that you're experimenting with sobriety for a while. If drinking is essential to the group, you may consider disconnecting from those people for a while—maybe that group is no longer a good match for your new lifestyle. Remember: Not everyone in your life is supposed to stay forever. Some people are with you for just a season.

In conclusion, right now you can't be swayed by others' questions or disapproval of your decision to be alcohol free. Your decision may remind them that they're drinking excessively or too frequently. Go easy on yourself and others; *don't take their negative comments in a personal way* or pay too much attention.

At the same time, stay open to the possibility that you're going to find new friends and/or connect with some of your existing friends *in new and healthier ways*. As you move through the fear zone and into the learning and growth zones, you'll be more whole and ready to take advantage of new connections and opportunities.

How to Feel Fun and Outgoing without Drinking

We can assure you that alcohol is not your personality, and it's *not* the drink that makes you feel fun, extroverted, or outgoing; *those aspects are inside you.* You can cultivate that way of connecting that involves being spontaneous, direct, present, going with the flow and knowing when it's the real you that feels a boundary or has some disinhibition.

In fact, being *alcohol free* gives you many more opportunities to feel *liberated from constraints in a controlled way.* This way, you can enjoy the freedom of being who you really are without the numbing effects of alcohol. Remember, there's power in staying true to yourself and being authentic in a consistent way, in a manner in which you're in control.

How to Participate in Social Events Where Drinking Is the Norm

Social life: As you know, drinking is such a part of our culture that if you don't drink, others often assume this is because you have or had a serious drinking problem. You could have a good explanation ready before heading to social events, but remember that you only need to share the information you're comfortable providing.

Holidays and celebrations: The happy moments that we share with family, friends, and colleagues can be ruined by alcohol, provoking problems, and taking away our chance to create good memories, because we don't remember the conversations we had while drinking in excess, or we cause turmoil or hurt feelings under the influence, or we suffer an ugly hangover the day after.

But going forward, all these scenarios are part of your past. *No more party drama*, at least not because of *your* drinking. Your celebrations will still be a lot of fun without alcohol, and you'll definitely appreciate your good decision when you wake up the next morning with no hangover or regrets. Sobriety makes it easier for us to experience all situations in a completely fresh way, rather than through a downgraded, diminished reality.

Prepare ahead for celebration and holiday occasions. For example, look at the menu in advance, bring your own alcohol-free drink, or stay at the gathering for a shorter time. If you can bring your own drink, you'll have a replacement beverage that you enjoy and no excuse to drink anything else. If going to a party or gathering makes you crave a drink, try to limit the time you'll be there, and maybe reward yourself with a good dessert or treat after. How you decide to handle holidays and celebrations will probably be connected to how close you are to the people inviting you, what the event is, and the group characteristics regarding drinking.

Be aware of your *past expectations* regarding alcohol and activate your *alcohol-free expectations*. If you used to always celebrate with a drink, new celebrations will be different, but as you start changing, you'll become more comfortable with the shift and feel better than before. This may seem impossible now, but stay with our method without questioning what's missing. With time, *you'll feel like you can do whatever you decide.*

How to Deal with Vacations

For many of us, alcoholic drinks have been an important part of vacations, trips, breaks, and staycations. When we decide not to drink, we may feel that we're *missing* something, that our holiday experience is not complete—until we realize that *the decision to be alcohol free is a win.*

An alcohol-free vacation keeps us fully present. You can enjoy the experience with more energy, without hangovers after a long night of drinking, and no alcohol-fuelled problems with those you're vacationing with. Waking up in the morning with a clear mind and more energy can create so many possibilities to explore places and connect with culture, people, history, and local foods—instead of sitting in a bar and drinking for hours.

Alcohol-Free Dating

Going on a date (especially a first date) can be challenging, because it's a unique one-to-one experience with expectations on both sides. As in other demanding situations, alcohol can be seen as "helpful," opening us up to vulnerability, empathy, and humor. But alcohol can also shadow our understanding of one another and the information we receive.

How can you manage being alcohol free and dating? Consider factors such as who you date, where you go, and when.

You could choose to meet or date people who are also *alcohol free*. Believe it or not, *becoming alcohol free is becoming more popular*, and there are a lot of people like you on this same journey.

Share only what you're comfortable disclosing about your decision to reconsider drinking or be alcohol free, while still being honest about yourself and your life. Don't worry too much about what the other person is going to think; this could be a good way to filter out those who won't be an appropriate partner in the long run. Choose the type of person who makes you feel understood and supported rather than minimizing of your decision.

You can plan dates and activities outside of bars and restaurants (go on a hike, explore a new part of the city, visit a museum or gallery, etc.). You might try meeting at a different time of the day when there are options other than a bar or restaurant.

Be creative, expand your horizons! Try a picnic, hiking, bowling, a class, or sunset in a park! Reconnect with previous interests that you might have forgotten because your relationship with alcohol was so absorbing. No more of those dates that push you to that edge where the only possibility is to drink.

If you do go to a bar or restaurant, what will you drink? Many places now have alcohol-free options beyond water or Diet Coke. You could try something more creative and sophisticated: a mocktail, a virgin cocktail, a nonalcoholic wine or beer.

The most important thing is that you *give some thought to all these factors and plan ahead* for how to manage situations that might make you feel awkward or pushed to drink again. Remember that without the numbing effects of alcohol, you'll be able to feel more deeply and authentically, especially when connecting with another person in the intense experience of dating. You have a lot to look forward to when it comes to alcohol-free dating!

Maintain a Connection with Significant Other or Reconstruct a Relationship

Becoming alcohol free can alter your personal relationship with your spouse, partner, or significant other. Routines and activities that you've had around drinking will change—whether cooking dinner together with a glass of wine, happy hour after work, trying a new bar on the weekend, finding a new wine or beer to enjoy together, going on a cruise or an all-inclusive vacation, etc. This change can affect your interactions, of course. Maybe drinking together has created intimacy and communication opportunities for you and your partner, but try to remember that it has certainly also led to *some or many problems along the way*.

During this transition *you need to put yourself and your life first.* Your relationship with yourself is primary; your relationships with others are secondary. You can't keep drinking in the same old way just to preserve your relationship or to make your significant other happy.

If drinking is something that you do with your partner and *both* of you want to quit, obviously it will take time and deep conversations to reach a point where you're both in agreement, feeling excited with the change, and prepared to support each other in areas of strength and weakness. Again, it usually takes some time and trial and error to get all these pieces flowing smoothly. Work together to find other interests and routines, to create a new environment that can replace alcohol and old drinking patterns.

It's possible that you won't both be on the same page, or not right away—maybe one of you wants to quit and the other doesn't. If only one of you wants to take a break from alcohol, give special attention to the reasons and consequences, and communicate, communicate, communicate. What can be done to support each other's respective decisions? This is a difficult question with many possible answers, because when one partner quits drinking, *the entire dynamic of the couple might change.* Looking for the positives and challenges and how to meet them is a sign of strength, and communication is key.

On the other hand, if being alcohol free creates a problem in your relationship, it may be because the relationship is a problem, and it will be wise to evaluate the foundation and future of your bond. Is *the relationship based solely or primarily on drinking together?* If so, this is a tremendous limitation if you have the intention to go further in the relationship.

Being alcohol free, especially if you decide to embark on this adventure together, can open new doors to what you can create together and give you greater possibilities than ever before in your personal relationship. The critical part to remember is that your life and decision to live better take priority over everything else.

Chapter 15: Guidance for Specific Challenges and Situations

Cope with Difficult Moments

People experiencing high stress and anxiety who drink usually report that they feel even more stressed and anxious the next day after drinking. Alcohol is a bad quality Band-Aid for stress and interpersonal problems. It may give you a few hours of comfort and coziness, but you'll pay the price the next day with cumulative consequences.

Our alcohol-soaked culture normalizes picking up a drink when difficult things happen as *the* way to forget about problems or stop worrying for the night or weekend. With an *alcohol-free* mind, you can see that this is a false premise. Drinking doesn't suppress or resolve trouble, but it does *limit our understanding and access to resources* to handle the situation.

Staying sober is a better way to deal with difficult moments so that you keep a clear mind, get better sleep, have less chance of experiencing regrets about what you said or did, and have more energy to resolve the problem.

Care for Yourself through the Times When You Used to Drink Alone

If you used to drink in solitude, your greatest *challenge* and *resource* now is simultaneously *you*! You are totally in charge of controlling your alcohol intake since you have *nobody around to pressure or encourage you one way or the other, or to check if you're drinking*. You are the only control you have.

Think about what will give you strength and resilience to meet this challenge. How can you plan and use your time differently? If you're used to drinking at home alone in the evenings, can you spend some time outside the home with no drinks around? For example, go to a workout class, try yoga, take a walk, learn a new hobby, meet up with a new group, get involved with your community, volunteer, etc. Change some of your solo routines completely, and look for enjoyable possibilities to replace drinking.

It's also essential that you make changes at home so that your space feels different and the old environmental or context cues to drink are no longer present in the same way. Move your furniture around, especially where you used to drink; declutter; redecorate; get a new plant; give away your favorite glass. Most importantly, remove all the alcohol—*no more booze at home.*

In conclusion, socializing and solitude are two key factors that influence drinking. You should consider how and where you socialize and how and where you spend time alone, your preferences, habits, and routines, and what changes you need to make to align with reconsidering your drinking and being alcohol free. Socializing and being alone both involve paying attention to external and internal influences and resources to support your decision.

If you're a social person and friends and get-togethers revolve around drinking, managing this change could present more external challenges. If you're used to drinking alone, you may need to mobilize more internal resources. In both cases, plan ahead, and use constructive options to replace old routines and desires.

If you were in the habit of drinking socially and alone, crossing the line in both these situations, you were at even greater risk of excessive drinking that can turn quickly into an alcohol disorder. Now you've made a brave change for you. It's going to take effort to build new habits to reach your goals. But you've gotten started, and as you continue to do the work, *your whole life will improve profoundly.*

Notes:

CHAPTER 16

GET PAST THE "JUST ONE DRINK" TRAP

I, Alicia, have been alcohol free for almost five years. On a recent flight to Miami to take a Caribbean cruise, the flight attendants served the business class passengers complimentary champagne. It seems that all sunny, beach vacations are paired with alcohol right from the start. The other passengers were accepting the drinks, and in the heat of the moment, my reaction went in two directions. I thought, *Oh, poor me, I don't drink anymore!* Then immediately after, *What about just one drink?*

The *"just one drink" trap* can appear at any moment. It might look *innocent*. Outwardly, you continue with whatever you're doing, but the *true focus* of your thoughts and feelings is *how good it would be if you could have a drink right now, just* one *drink*.

The tricky part is that, usually, there's nobody there to say that you can or can't drink. *You're the one confronting your own urges in a very personal way,* using your own tools and resources and all you've learned from getting past your comfort zone, going through the fear and learning zones, and consolidating your growth.

"I know what will happen if I have 'just one drink': I'm going to tell myself, 'It's just one drink. Surely, I've learned how to moderate my drinking by now. Everyone else seems like they're having fun. Why can't I? Why not? What's the harm? I swear, I'll have just one.'" —Marlene

Just *thinking* like Marlene will *build up a desire to drink*. You start trying to decide what to do and bargaining with yourself. But all's not fair in this war, because on one side is your desire to maintain your alcohol-free identity, and on the other side is your emotional self that *acts mainly by impulse*. Another component is peer interaction and if your friends who drink are pressuring you in that direction. Eventually, *you could convince yourself that there's no harm in just one glass of your favorite wine.*

This could happen in any *personal situation*, like celebrations, breakups, difficult moments, a night alone at home, a stressful day, during a date night; and at *family or social events*, such as graduations, weddings, vacations, meals, and holidays. The list of where the "just one drink" trap can appear is endless. You can count on it popping up efficiently and consistently during the highs and lows of life.

We'll present some characteristics and cases of these different situations, so that you can identify which are more prevalent in your life and develop some tools to respond.

Holidays and Celebrations

"After Dry January, a close friend invited me to attend her wedding. My experience of being sober for thirty days was difficult but positive, and I was seriously considering quitting forever. That was a significant change in my thinking, since I'd always considered sober people boring.

Chapter 16: Get Past the "Just One Drink" Trap

"The wedding reception was last weekend, and I had every intention of not drinking. When I could finally sit down and relax after going around and greeting friends, I suddenly thought: 'I'll have just one drink.' Many acquaintances had asked me why I wasn't drinking, and I just felt that I needed to be like them, to feel 'normal' on this occasion. I felt like I was going against societal norms, like I was an embarrassment by not drinking. You know how it is, people assume you've had a huge alcohol problem if you don't drink at a wedding.

"Well, even though I struggled with myself, with societal expectations, with that party and celebrations in general, I was able to return to my center and my decision to live alcohol free. I didn't have that 'one drink.' I felt proud and brave, a real badass." —Angela

Holidays and celebrations are times of closeness with the special people in our lives, times to enjoy their company, to be joyous, to be happy together for an occasion. *We live in a drinking society,* and because of that, whether the celebration is an intimate event, a work party, family get-together, holiday, graduation, or a splendid wedding, alcohol is typically an essential element of the occasion. Gatherings or celebrations can also be a time of social anxiety for many, and alcohol reduces social inhibition, promoting relaxation and enjoyment, so drinking can be important for this reason, too.

We've been conditioned to think that special celebrations *must* have alcoholic drinks. Therefore, being alcohol-free and rejecting this essential element could cause confusion, distrust, mistrust, suspicion, and other adverse reactions, as if you were from another planet or, worse, a current or former alcoholic.

However, if you have even *just one drink*, you're going to be unhappy about that choice for at least two reasons:

1. Just one drink will not satisfy you. End of story. You'll need a second one and maybe a third. Can you imagine how you'll feel the next morning?
2. Having just one drink shows lack of respect for your decision to not drink. Disrespecting yourself is going to affect your self-confidence and self-esteem.

Self-confidence and self-esteem are the motors of the self, and if these are running low, you're going *to doubt yourself*, feeling that you aren't good enough. This can affect your decision to be alcohol free as well as any other goals you've set your sights on, because with low self-esteem, you're *less likely to believe in yourself*.

First Dates

"I'm in my early thirties and single again. Almost all my friends are in serious relationships. I broke up with my ex, Randy, because we had big differences in our lifestyles and finally decided to go our separate ways. After years of drinking excessively, first during college and later with my friends during weekends at the local brewery and drinking for hours, one of the few things on which I agreed with Randy was to take a break from alcohol. It was easy to do it together, initially. But after a few months, Randy wanted to use alcohol again, and I wanted to stay alcohol free, so this led to a lot of changes for us, and eventually, we ended our relationship.

"I really want to settle down with someone, so I've been dating again. I met Martin on a dating app. We've been texting a lot and have talked over the phone several times, so I feel I know him pretty

Chapter 16: Get Past the "Just One Drink" Trap

well. We're planning to meet up in person, and Martin suggested having dinner together. Dinners on the first date come with drinks, so I've been thinking, after being alcohol free for seventeen months, is having just one drink okay? I don't know what to do. If I don't drink, he might think that I'm weird or an alcoholic. If I do drink, I'd feel I don't respect myself and my decision to be sober and that I'll go back to square one." —Serena

This may feel like a complicated situation, given the pervasiveness of alcohol culture. In many social circles, a typical pattern for first dates is to have two drinks with dinner. In order to confront this contradictory situation positively, think about the following:

- On the one side, you have the cultural premise that dates often happen at bars or restaurants. Besides going along with what seems customary, meeting in those places can also be convenient for another reason: the anxiety of meeting or dating a new person can be lessened with a couple of drinks. You might wonder, *will the other person feel comfortable and interested in a relationship with me if we can't drink together?*
- On the other side is your reality of being alcohol free—and an important question: *How are you going to be comfortable with and true to yourself?*

Even if you know that the "just one drink" card is not the answer, you might feel that it's okay to make an exception in this particular circumstance *to show that you're "normal."* But it's especially in this specific circumstance that the "just one drink" card is a trap.

Given the potential for the intensely personal experiences and feelings of a first date, our best advice is to *be authentic and sincere,* with yourself first of all, and in showing the real you to the other person. Be careful about creating false expectations. We can't control how other people act, react, or handle relationships. But we can and should take control of our actions and decisions. It's your right and responsibility *to respect yourself first, to put yourself in first place.*

Breakups

"*A mutual friend introduced me to Joseph. We ended up having really intense chemistry and started seeing each other the same week. We both had been married and divorced before. Even though we said we didn't want to rush because of our previous experiences, we were totally into each other. We started spending weekends together, then went on some short trips, and our casual dating quickly became a real relationship.*

"*After six months, Joseph started to change. He was 'busy,' 'tired,' or 'sick,' and most of our plans had to be postponed. He delayed answering my texts, and when he did answer, he was terse or in a hurry.*

"*Long story short: I asked Joseph what was going on and if we could talk. He said that even though we had good chemistry, he thought there was nothing else to justify continuing our relationship since we had different lifestyles. He felt our personalities weren't a good match.*

"*I returned to my apartment alone after that final talk. Even though I'd spent more than two years being alcohol free, I thought about having just one drink to deal with this unbelievable breakup.*"
—Kylee

If you've faced a situation like Kylee's, thinking about playing the "just one drink" card is understandable. But it's *not going to add solutions to the situation.* Moreover, you'll be giving someone else the power to take away not only your sobriety but also a promising future. In a relationship, you might have fifty percent of the power; in your sobriety, you have one hundred percent of the command. *So, own it. Don't give it away.*

Life Problems

"I've worked very hard for my career and future. My spouse and I don't have children, and consequently, we've had a lot of freedom. We both are alcohol free and have enjoyed being sober and the many opportunities this has given us.

"Recently, I went to the doctor for my annual physical. A few days later, I got a message urging me to see the doctor again. I received shocking news that I had breast cancer and most likely needed surgery and chemotherapy. More studies were done, and the diagnosis was confirmed. We were appalled. I felt like our future and everything I've worked for was going to be compromised. We returned home, and I thought about having a drink for the first time in three years." —Julia

When problems or difficult situations impact us, it's normal to seek comfort and to want to forget challenging circumstances, at least for a while. "Just one drink" can appear to be an ideal "solution" for two reasons. First, it can numb us by relaxing our thoughts and worries; and second, it can give us an overly optimistic view of the situation, at least for a while.

In reality, the "just one drink" card is not effective in situations where you must be engaged on all levels to find resources and solutions and not worsen an already challenging situation. *Numbing yourself will be to your detriment.* In difficult times, it's even more important to connect with the friends, activities, and coping strategies you've developed to replace your relationship with alcohol.

Boredom

> "I'm forty-five and have been married for almost twenty years. Our son just left for college, so for the first time since our twenties, my husband and I are by ourselves. In the past, I had a group of friends with whom I used to drink, but since I quit drinking, I don't see them as often. I had to make a decision to take a break from that scene, because I was drinking in excess every day. I realized that I wasn't far from being an alcoholic, and I got really scared. It was a difficult decision but worth it.
>
> "A few weeks after I stopped drinking, I started to feel good, with more energy. I slept better and lost some weight, which was wonderful! But I was also distanced from my usual social group. There were changes in my routine with my husband, too. One of our times to connect was in the evenings; we'd sit on our deck with a couple of drinks and talk. Those were special moments. I feel much better now that I'm not drinking, but I'm lonely and bored to death. Sometimes I feel that just one drink with my friends or my husband is all I need to feel better." —Nellie

Boredom can be a pivotal factor when it comes to the risk of relapse and must be considered seriously. Lots of people drink because they're bored. Remember the quote, *"An idle mind is the devil's playground"?* When you're in that space, anything other than being bored is appealing, and alcohol looks attractive and is often easily accessible! You remember only the "fun times" and not the alcohol-induced poor sleep, hangovers, or headaches the next morning. The "just one drink" card is an accessible resource, and you feel an urgency to have just one drink. Alcohol gives some momentary relief, but after a short time, it's tremendously inefficient.

Boredom often is a leading factor in determining relapse. We think we have the right to choose something that takes us away from feeling bored.—We do, but it doesn't have to be alcohol. Don't give that old, seductive, destructive lover your power.

The strength to respond to boredom comes from sitting with that feeling, going inside ourselves to see or discover our predispositions, inclinations, preferences, and likings. From there, we can choose new routines, activities, or hobbies that match what really matters to us. This is a powerful choice, because it moves you in the direction of your motivations, growth, and pleasure. It requires determination, dedication, and effort, but it will allow you *to break the cycle of boredom and its consequences in successful and joyful ways.* What a gift to have time to try something new, learn a new skill, and improve your life!

In conclusion, as with any decision in life, we should look at the different factors and sides:

1. In thinking about playing the "just one drink" card, we're looking at a possibility: *If I drink, I might enjoy momentary satisfaction, company, and fun.* But there's another consideration, that drinking has a price: *I might have problems with controlling how much I decide to drink during this event or after. My alcohol-free identity is going to be affected, along with my self-esteem and confidence.*

2. The decision to not drink *may* take away a particular type of short-term enjoyment, but it also protects you from falling back into the negative vicious cycle from which you've worked hard to be free. *If I don't drink, I'll gain the profound benefits of sobriety. I'll be able to access enjoyment and experiences I wouldn't have had if I hadn't persevered with being alcohol free.*

It's a good idea to make a list of the related pros and cons. What will you choose in your search for the best option?

If you resist the temptation of "just one drink" and stay strong, in a short time you'll experience some peace with yourself and the situation you've chosen. This will increase your sense of self-worth and happiness that comes from *following through with what you've decided for your life*; and it will decrease the chance of getting into complications.

Gradually, you'll discover that the attractive effects you've attributed to alcohol are likely due to *genuine but perhaps unknown or underdeveloped aspects of yourself* that you can now discover and develop as you live in your new alcohol-free identity. Say, for instance, that you've felt more fun, free, social, and empathetic when drinking. You can be confident that these qualities come from *you*, not from a glass of wine. *It will be an extraordinary adventure to go deeply into yourself, to uncover and cultivate these treasured qualities and give them full expression.* These gems are part of your personality, maybe not yet wholly familiar to you, but absolutely *not part of the drink.*

Please understand that sobriety means no drinking, clear and straightforward. The "just one drink" card is fallacious and deceptive. It seems innocent, but using this card is going to take you away from your goals and new alcohol-free identity. If you give a hand to your drink, it will take your entire arm. *One drink is hardly ever "just one drink."*

At the end of the day, you know that alcohol is a drug that provokes addiction, and there's no escape. It could take one year or twenty, but, if you were to get back into or continue drinking, eventually you would end up with an alcohol disorder and face major consequences. If you were to start drinking again because of situations and circumstances—just one drink today at a party, another tomorrow because you're stressed out—slowly you'll *go back to the same amount of alcohol you were drinking when you began this journey.* The "one drink" card seems innocent, but if you use it, you'll find yourself confronting internal and external factors with minimal possibilities of winning.

The best answer is NO. Stay away from the "just one drink" trap. *Stand focused and strong in your new alcohol-free life.*

Notes:

CHAPTER 17

BUILD AN ALCOHOL-FREE IDENTITY, THE KEY TO FREEDOM

Here's another million-dollar question: *How do you develop a new personal identity centered on being alcohol free?*

When we take time to get curious about our drinking identity and peel back the layers of our "beliefs" and "personal characteristics" (see Chapter 6), we'll usually find that these elements are actually related to social norms and customs we've learned consciously or subconsciously. Drinking norms and an alcohol-oriented identity are *not* inherently part of our true self.

When we decide to free ourselves from something—our drinking identity, in this case—that has become part of how we see ourselves or perceive others see us, we often find ourselves grieving for, or missing, that part of our self and the related behaviors, people, places, and routines that supported this aspect of our identity. Now we've decided to change, to leave that context, that part of us, behind, but it's the hardest part, because we haven't fully established our new norms and behaviors yet. We're not settled yet in our new sense of self. We're doing all this work based on *just our decision and willpower.*

In addition, as you know, many things connected to drinking are considered positive in our society. Being sober is thought to suggest the opposite: lacking self-control; being dull, uninteresting, judgmental, distrustful, a former alcoholic—all negatives. So, you must be careful with your mindset (your attitude), because if you take in others' comments and opinions about being sober without question, you're likely to think that you're going to *lose* (not gain) and miss out on friendships, family times, and fun in general.

The first step to developing a personal identity centered on being alcohol free is to *disconnect from that old drinking identity*. You may feel empty or lonely in the early stages of making this change, thinking that *it's you against this big bad world*. It *is* a huge challenge, because we make this decision alone—it comes from deep within yourself—without knowing exactly what we're going to do with our social life, at home, or during the times when we always used to drink; without knowing how we'll feel living an alcohol-free life. However, never forget that you have powerful tools and inner resources at your disposal, starting with your willpower, confidence, and self-esteem, to build up this new part of your identity that is alcohol free.

Everyone who has decided to be alcohol free, including us, has experienced this difficult process where we go from feeling like we have a *socially accepted awesome drinking identity* to a *weird, disconnected sense of self*, without anything solid to plant our feet on yet, while also fielding questions and even judgment and criticism from family members, friends, and acquaintances.

Our identity is both *personally and socially informed*. It's common to face an *identity crisis* when you go through life transitions. It's probable that you will experience this type of crisis in the process of becoming alcohol free. Use the information about the stages of grief for support.

Remember that you don't need to wait to feel "motivated" or "different" to change. Even if you don't always "feel motivated," keep practicing your new habits and routines. When you do things differently, because you want to and know that it's right for you, feelings and thoughts of motivation usually kick in. Let your new positive, healthier, wiser behaviors lead the way. Act as though you're motivated, and your thoughts and feelings will follow. Know that if you do the work, and stick to your goal, your identity will *grow, transform, evolve, and expand* like never before. You will gain so much in exchange for letting go of your drink.

Changes and Challenges in Developing an Alcohol-Free Identity

What are some of the changes and challenges you can expect as you develop an alcohol-free identity?

"I'm a lawyer and married, with two kids in college, and a husband that respects me—essentially because I bring more money to the table than him. My job is intense, and the way I relax is by drinking with colleagues and friends after work. At the end of a hard day, and after a lot of stressful moments and introspection as to whether I did well with the cases I'm handling, I like to sit down for a happy hour and be myself. I feel free, easygoing, excited. I love feeling like this.

"The problem is that this identity lasts a short time; then a different aspect of my personality appears: controlling, demanding, hard to please, and sometimes even rude. But this second part doesn't count. I'm always looking forward to the positive way I feel during the first two drinks; I'm addicted to that experience, even if it lasts just a short time.

> *"I'm starting to think about becoming alcohol free, but this is the major obstacle: Who would I be if I decide not to drink? The good or the bad? Who am I really? I wonder if I'll be a totally different person when sober. And what about my friends? Will they avoid and reject me? Will they connect with my alcohol-free personality? Maybe nobody will want to be around me if I become sober."* —Ruby

When you were a *social drinker*, you were part of groups that gathered in bars or restaurants or each other's homes to drink. Being a member of a drinking culture brings connection, a sense of self, and belonging to a group(s). This social part of our drinking identity can become so ingrained that it's difficult to break away, because it feels like a loss. Additionally, our friends or family may not understand, or may even be upset by our change. Consequently, your social network may decrease abruptly; you may need to be prepared to go it alone and get comfortable hanging out with yourself until you find a new tribe.

If you used *to drink alone*, becoming alcohol free can be a fast track to discovering who you really are away from the effects of alcohol. Honor and use this time to return to and connect with yourself and whatever you're experiencing—the good, the bad, and the ugly. Drinking has kept you in a comfort zone with your preferred way of dealing with your everyday (having drinks at the end of each day by yourself), removing other possibilities and confining you to *a downgraded reality*. Many things at home will have to change as you go through this process. You'll need to find new positive routines and things you like to do to fill the times when you used to drink.

Chapter 17: Build an Alcohol-Free Identity, the Key to Freedom

"One year ago, I fell ill and was taken to the hospital. When they released me and sent me home, I was told I shouldn't drink for the next three months due to the medication I had to take. After a few days, I started missing drinking in the evenings. I used to sit in my garden with a drink and reflect on the day and my plans, ideas, etc.

"When I considered staying sober forever, my thoughts and feelings were about how to adjust to life without alcohol, how I was going to be, and how to replace those good moments. Drinking was absolutely related to my identity and lifestyle. I realized how strong the drinking habit can be, but I also recognized that my identity certainly could develop along richer and more brilliant roads.

"I feel that I'm changing as time goes by. It's not easy, but I'm finding a new part of me that I really like. Also, I'm noticing that I have more time, money, and a clear mind the next day!" —Pamela

As you can see, your drinking identity may have been deeply rooted in your personal and social realities. These social and personal elements may also be the exact things that you have to work through in becoming sober. The only way to break free is through *personal work and concrete actions*. You might consider the following steps:

- Stay away from drinking groups and friends, at least until you feel at peace with yourself and with your decision to take a break from alcohol. We aren't saying that you shouldn't hang out with your people, but do set boundaries and avoid situations that tempt you to drink. Instead of hanging out at a restaurant or a bar, suggest meeting up for an activity that does not require drinking.
- Read books and articles, watch documentaries and TV series about the consequences of drinking.

- Read inspirational stories to find ideas for building your new alcohol-free identity.
- Follow a motivational speaker with a clear message that resonates with this stage of your life.
- Calculate how much money you're saving each week and month by not buying alcohol. Put it toward something you want or would like to do that you weren't able to afford before (a hobby, travel, etc.). Now you can!
- Look for new alcohol-free connections and sober social groups and enjoy their company, tips, routines, and stories. Through these groups, you'll discover and connect with new ideas, activities, alcohol-free drinks, places, hobbies, and ways of staying social while living alcohol free.
- Learn how to deal with problems and pressures effectively instead of repressing and trying to forget them through drinking.
- Use trial and error, find what works for you and what doesn't. Try new things, and see how you feel. *Take what you want; leave what doesn't work*.
- Prepare in advance for situations that would make you feel inclined to drink.

Whether you drink with others or in solitude, when you become alcohol free, your sense of self changes. Several forces might oppose your becoming sober, and you have to go through some difficult moments, as you adapt to living without alcohol. This is the time to find yourself in this new reality, to *build a new identity that doesn't need alcohol,* and to live accordingly, recognizing and responding to new realities.

Sometimes this process includes becoming aware of problems or areas you were previously unaware of or avoiding that now require your attention. It can also involve becoming aware of interests and strengths you hadn't been able to recognize before. Maybe this is the first opportunity you have to focus on *you*, the *real you*, without the artificially enhanced or numb feelings provoked by alcohol.

As you redefine and clarify who you are, give yourself time and freedom to build and explore your alcohol-free identity. Focus on what you truly value in yourself and in your surroundings:

- *In yourself*: What are your strengths? What do you like about yourself? What motivates you? What do you enjoy? What actions and activities promote personal growth? How can you contribute to others? Get to know this emerging you.
- *In your surroundings*: What new opportunities are here? (This includes in relationships, personal interests, work, hobbies, new habits, etc.)

In conclusion, by making this change to develop an alcohol-free identity, *you set yourself free*. Instead of being swept along by societal conditions, your eyes and mind are open and clear to your new reality. You're looking inside yourself and around you, appreciating your journey, even the difficult days, because it brings change and growth. *This time and this process are gifts life is offering you, and you are accepting them*!

Becoming alcohol free is like *illuminating a room*. Before you could see only a couple of feet around you, but now you can see the whole room and appreciate the totality of this wonderful space, with paintings, colors, decorations, comforts, and elements that were previously hidden in the darkness.

This bright room is your new identity. The new alcohol-free you.

Notes:

CHAPTER 18

DESIGN YOUR BRIGHT FUTURE

Now that you've liberated yourself from your previous alcohol-centered lifestyle, you may have a better idea of who you were before your relationship with alcohol started, and the *potential that is within and around you* as you continue your journey of inner exploration and growth. This is an exciting and thrilling time for you to connect or reconnect with yourself, to become grounded in *your real identity*, who you are in this moment, and *what you want for your future*.

The starting point for a happy life is connecting to our authentic self; keeping things real; no longer hiding behind appearances, pretending to be more or better than we are. Pay attention to feelings of not being good enough, self-blame, or judgment from others. Practice self-compassion. Remind yourself of the value of going step by step to build a strong foundation. This time can be an incredible experience and opportunity to grow, focusing on your essence, and inspiring others to also live an authentic life, true to themselves. Now is when you can start *visualizing an exciting time to come and begin to build this future for yourself.*

Looking forward to the future with eager anticipation may be a new experience. When you used to drink, thinking about the future might have been scary, because your reactions were based on external, societal expectations and conditions. Your "vision" about the future may have been limited and primarily focused on whether you were crossing the line; if you were going to become an alcoholic; experiencing the flash of clarity during early mornings or when you were unable to sleep in the middle of the night; feeling you didn't have the willpower to make a change, followed by feelings of denial, shame, and low self-esteem.—A vicious cycle. It may have seemed that there was no point to thinking ahead or trying to change. It may have been painful even to contemplate the future, because you didn't know how to break free from that destructive lover, your drink. But no more! You have freed yourself from this negative dependence, and what's ahead for you is bright and magnificent.

To open to this exciting adventure, take time to be curious about yourself and your surroundings: *What type of future do you want? What do you value the most? Who do you want to be on a consistent basis? What would you like to do? What is your focus? What feelings do you want to have on a regular basis? Who can support you? What and who do you need to leave behind?*

- With the greater clarity you have from leaving alcohol behind and caring for your inner life, you can have deeper and more honest realizations about your emotions and thoughts. Reflect on your authentic personal attributes and characteristics, your values, what matters to you in this stage of your life. Who is the real you, and how do you want to live? What makes you happy?
- Think about your social reality, starting with your family, friends, coworkers; look at past and current experiences and situations. Who is going to stay and where do you need to make changes in your relationships? Remember that not everyone is supposed to stay in our lives forever. Who needs to be in your life? Are there

people whose presence and relationships are toxic and no longer healthy for you? What steps will you take?

By exploring and reconnecting to these elements of your relationship to yourself and with others, based on where and who you are today, you can open to what you want in your future. What values, interests, and priorities do you want to consider?

During this time of reflection and visioning, you may want to reconnect with your social reality gradually and selectively. *Take it easy,* because *you are a different person* now, and your (former) drinking friends and social groups may not be okay with you and your decision and changes. *They* may not have changed, and so they may not like or relate to how much you have grown. *Be gentle with yourself and with others, and stay true to your convictions.* Some relationships will continue over time; others will deteriorate, and that's okay.

It's important to do this work gradually, step by step. You don't have to puzzle out your magnificent future straightaway. Devote time to exploring your possibilities and opportunities; see what matches your desires and how, and what resources you have or can develop. This period requires personal work and involves a great deal of fun and creativity.

"Drinking was part of my identity for many years, with vodka being my partner of choice during good times and bad days. Everything in my life was connected to drinking, whether I was at home alone or with my partner, after work with my coworkers, in social groups with my dear friends and acquaintances, and during vacations, celebrations, and holidays. Not one aspect of my life was sober.

"At that point, I didn't want to think about my future. I feared what could happen if I continued drinking that way. Many of my friends

already had problems related to drinking, like tremors in their hands, a nasty divorce provoked by excessive drinking, or a DWI.

"When I decided to do a Dry January, I found myself missing the drink and all its related effects. It was like longing for a lost friend! It took me a while to start thinking it was a good idea to quit. Could I actually do this, not just for a month but for forever? I started to have compassion for myself and thinking that I deserved a better future. That helped me work through the process.

"It took a lot of work to leave that reality and to question myself about my real identity and what I wanted for the future. It took me time to realize that it was safe to let myself think about the future because there could be good ahead, and I was worthy of positive experiences, and not just sad outcomes from overdrinking. Eventually, it became exciting to anticipate what I could be and do.

"Gradually, I started finding things that motivated me and gave me purpose. The best part was that a new me was developing. I've become unstoppable in reaching my new goals. I enjoy my progress in this new stage of my life, and I'm much happier than before." —Melissa

Becoming alcohol free is a time of *personal growth, discovering a vision for your future, and building step by step toward that* by:

- *Connecting with strengths that have been lying dormant*, whether these are existing strengths from your life so far, or strengths you've newly identified or are starting to build up.
- *Finding your purpose and motivation for an attractive future*. What could be your new role in life? Who will be with you on this journey? What's your main focus? What excites you?
- *Repairing or deepening essential relationships*; gaining confidence and skills to manage past difficulties, make amends, end rela-

tionships that are no longer healthy, and keep doing your best in the present.

Taking these steps will give you balance, happiness, and confidence today and in your exciting future. It's up to you *to get up and act* with determination and purpose, considering your hopes and desires.

Our society's normalization and idealization of drinking has ruined so many lives. Alcohol is ingrained in all aspects of our existence, and that makes breaking free from the drinking habit extra difficult. But it's a change that's a hundred percent possible, extremely positive, and rewarding.

You've already recognized and taken on the challenge of *making a wiser choice*, accepting that it requires a positive mindset and determination. Instead of feeling scared about the future or entertaining regrets about what you did or said while you were drinking, you're now focused on the discovery process ahead, which is constructive and uplifting. You've decided to deal with *short-term pain* in order to gain *long-term pleasure* and open yourself to a *positive future full of possibilities*.

"Becoming alcohol free liberated and redefined me and my life in ways I couldn't have imagined before! I'm better, more open, more intentional, and of course, more fun, all because I'm clear-minded, full of energy, and happier now. I found a new way to live, I have joy and the possibility to grow and decide what I want. I'm no longer in a constant state of worry about what could happen with my life if I continued drinking as I was. I hardly recognize myself as the person I was one year ago. I had my schedule and managed my responsibilities, but my life revolved around the anticipation of my 'reward'—my drinks—at the end of the day. Now I can focus on areas in my life that I can improve, projects for my present, goals for my future, and even spiritual things that I formerly didn't pay much attention to." —Grace

You can create an extraordinary life if you decide to become alcohol free. As you begin to experience the cumulative positives of quitting alcohol and the surprise of the incredible reality that you're already living or will be experiencing soon, a new you is blossoming. *You're constructing a magnificent future. You're now in charge of your life.*

Notes:

CHAPTER 19

THE TRIPOD OF SELF-LOVE, IDENTITY, AND A BRIGHT FUTURE

Sarah, a successful entrepreneur in her early fifties, was part of exciting social and professional circles. Since college, she had used alcohol to cope with the pressures of her demanding career. She started crossing the line at one point, primarily when she drank by herself. The extent of her alcohol use was a secret to her social circle, her fiancé, and even herself. She began having problems in her relationships and with close friends and found herself having to work double-time to maintain her business reputation as productive, efficient, and professional. That was difficult since her energy was low, especially in the mornings when the most critical decision-making occurred.

One day, out of the blue, she decided she didn't want to continue this downward spiral and quit drinking. *This change kickstarted a positive cycle connecting her identity, self-love, and bright compelling future.*

- She noticed a change in her identity. She went from perceiving herself as weak and incapable, especially after evenings spent drinking, to a sense of possibility—not only in her career but

- also in other personal interests, such as hobbies and service to her community. This energized her, and her sense of self grew as she maintained her decision to be sober.
- With her identity refreshed and strengthened, she started looking at her future differently. Instead of concentrating exclusively on her high-stress job, she started creating new paths in her personal and professional life. Sarah began to go on cultural trips, leading to interactions with diverse communities. She mentored young women who wanted to build a career. Also, she solidified her committed relationship with her fiancé.
- With her reconnection to an expanded, exciting future that grew out of her renewed identity, she became more aware and appreciative of her possibilities and determination. As a result of being able to quit alcohol, Sarah nurtured a newfound sense of self-love and self-appreciation and valued her resilience. This further enhanced her self-perception, completing the loop and starting its next iteration. *Sarah had figured out how to put the tripod to work for her.*

Quitting alcohol was a turning point in Sarah's life. It allowed her to better manage emotional issues and practical decisions related to her personal interests. That led her to reconnect with and strengthen her identity, from which she could start thinking of new goals to build her future and make it an exciting, fulfilling one. In turn, her self-love was expanded, providing her hope and a sense of purpose. A foundation of self-love continued to boost her positive sense of self and bright future.

When you decide to quit alcohol, you are reconnecting with your true self to create a *new or revitalized identity* that separates you from your old drinking personality. Under that identity, you were full of shame, guilt, low self-confidence, and fears about your future. When you decided to take care of yourself, take control, and reduce your drinking, you began claiming your alcohol-free identity, clearing off the rubble of the ruin and destruction drinking creates. Now, you're starting to perceive yourself differently in relation to your increased self-worth. You define yourself based on the positive changes you have made in your life. *Understanding how you can build up your new alcohol-free identity and increase your self-love will improve your future and happiness decisively.*

Identity and self-love are closely related. *Self-love* includes accepting who you are, treating yourself well; taking care of your body, mind, and soul; standing up for yourself; believing you can do anything you decide to do; and remembering that all the resources you need start from within you. Self-love is a journey with ups and downs; it requires practice, work, and opening to the possibilities of loving ourselves, loving others, and feeling loved.

Self-love isn't selfishness or greed. You are the person with whom you will have a lifelong relationship. So, you are the first person you need to love, the first person you have to take care of before everyone else. You have to become your own best friend. Learning to love yourself, to befriend yourself, to be kind to yourself is essential to your growth and contentment, and it boosts you in supporting and loving others. Love and open-heartedness toward yourself will help you create the solid foundation you can trust and build from to develop strengths and talents.

When we're optimistic about ourselves, we'll also be more open to investing in our well-being and connecting with a *compelling future*—just the opposite of what you felt before. When you were drinking, the future was frightening, filled with the real risks of losing your health, relationships, and career. The feeling of being unable to control your drinking might have made you think that you weren't good enough, that you were worthless, that you had no future. The beliefs and feelings about self that stem from drinking all lead to negatives, not to mention the multiple other issues that drinking can cause.

Trusting and investing in your well-being will lead you to a place of calmness and recognition of your potential to build a better you, fulfilling relationships, and an improved career. You'll have energy and clarity to start planning exciting new things and following goals with a positive mindset and self-love; you'll get the motivation to build a stimulating future. Self-love acts as a promoter of personal growth and restoration, giving the motivation for better times to come.

You've crossed a bridge and are now standing across from where you were before—in a place where your identity was linked to a situation that didn't allow you to grow, your future was scary, and your low self-love negatively affected your life, making you drink more and more, and sabotaging any effort to get better. Loving yourself first is a positive catalyst to making and sustaining change in your life.

> *"My journey from overdrinking almost every day to quitting and living alcohol free has changed me. I'd battled with alcohol since my late twenties, so this had taken a lot of my life. In all those years, I'd lost sight of my real identity and hopefulness for the future. Self-love was nonexistent—moreover, I didn't trust myself anymore, and sometimes I hated myself for not being able to control my drinking, an addiction that slowly damaged me, my job, and my relationship with my soulmate.*
>
> *"I hit rock bottom after a heartbreaking experience when my husband asked to part ways. He was done with me and my drinking. That shocked me. I felt I couldn't continue my alcohol habit; something had to change. I faced my fears, and with determination, I started looking for help. First, I read a book. At that time, I was so ashamed*

of myself that I didn't want anybody to know my secret. Reading was something I could do privately, on my own.

"I began to heal and reconnect with my true identity. I continued to read self-help books in the evenings, the time I'd previously used to drink the most. I explored new and old interests, like drawing and painting, a hobby that I had once enjoyed but abandoned due to my negative habits. Reading and creating art became strong sources of comfort, self-expression, and a way to connect with and help others. Reconnecting with these passions gave me an intense sense of purpose. I feel more alive now than I have in a long time.

"Learning to love myself again was a challenging but central part of my healing. Slowly, I'm letting go of the guilt and shame that I had for so many years while I drank. Drinking affected my self-esteem, worth, and confidence to go after positive goals. Practicing self-compassion allowed me to rebuild my self-love and start being comfortable with the person I am today and who I'm becoming. It's led to being more hopeful about my future. I keep setting goals for myself as I continue transforming my life in ways that were unimaginable to me before.

"Quitting the horrible habit of drinking improved my mental and physical health. I started working out again. Not only is my body getting leaner, but I also feel stronger and calmer. These days, I like to share my story, which proves that change is possible and that even in difficult situations, there's hope for a happier tomorrow." —Ruth

Remember, you owe care to yourself first before anyone else. You are your first priority in this life. Everything else comes after you. The more energy you have, the more you can give to others. *This is your time to focus on your happiness, your goals, your future, your relationships—to focus on you. Who do you want to become?*

Crossing the Line Can Disrupt the Loop of Self-Love, Identity, and a Bright Future

Crossing the line can disrupt the positive loop of self-love, identity, and a compelling future through two influential ways: 1) *Alcohol is a physical and psychological depressor*, and 2) *The habit of drinking can promote health problems and weight gain*. Let's look at these two points in detail:

1. Disruption of the loop because of the depressor effect of alcohol: Let's say we drink every night and wake up tired every day. Alcohol affects how we see ourselves and the way we think about and approach our goals and future.

Identity: The use of alcohol can diminish a person's identity, disconnecting them from their true self, values, and goals.

Self-love: Since using alcohol can exacerbate feelings of depression and sadness, drinking can intensify self-questioning and a lack of self-compassion, deteriorating the possibility of accessing kinder (and healthier) ways to cope.

The Future: Alcohol is a depressant, and drinking can affect an individual's vision of the future. When we feel down emotionally, our future appears scary and monotonous, rather than exciting and energizing, powered by a clear vision, and guided by personal growth and positive goals.

In summary, understanding that alcohol is a depressant helps us to recognize how drinking can affect the way we see ourselves, our goals and choices; and limits the path to a positive way of living. Being alcohol free cuts through that depressive noise and baggage, allowing us to reconnect with our sense of self, self-love, real identity, and a compelling future.

2. Disruption of the loop because of alcohol-induced weight gain: Women already experience a lot of societal pressure and messaging that pushes fear, stigma, and judgment regarding weight and appearance. In addition to these pressures, alcohol can cause weight gain, which can be connected to a loss of positive self-perception and external image. Loss of positive self-identity can affect self-worth and what we expect and pursue in the future.

Identity: Alcohol's effect on weight can influence an individual's sense of self and lead to feelings of low self-esteem and poor body image. If individuals gain extra weight from alcohol use, they may lose self-confidence and face negative social stereotypes related to being overweight.

Self-love: Caring for one's physical and emotional well-being is part of self-love. Not taking into consideration that alcohol can lead to weight gain and changes in personal image, individuals might find themselves suddenly feeling lower confidence, affecting their self-love.

The Future: The impact of weight gain could limit an individual's vision of their future and what's possible in personal, social, and career opportunities. When we are not in tune with our bodies, our future may seem scary since we tend to limit ourselves when our body image does not match with how we want to look.

In summary, the connection between alcohol and weight gain can affect how individuals perceive themselves, align with their goals, and envision a stimulating future. So, it is essential to consider what is healthy and suitable to eat and drink as part of your self-care. *This could be a strong force for constructive change and healing.*

Choosing an Identity

When we drink often, and our lives revolve around our next drink, we become a heavy drinker, a functioning alcoholic; or, in later stages, a chronic-severe alcoholic. Even if we don't recognize consciously that we're becoming an alcoholic, subconsciously, we know that we're misusing alcohol at some level, and this informs our sense of self. It follows *that we would then identify ourselves, privately or publicly, as a drinker, heavy drinker, functioning alcoholic, drunk, or alcoholic.*

This is key because our identity is essential and determines the *choices* we make and the *results* we get. For example, a person whose actions identify them as a heavy drinker lives an entirely different life from someone who identifies as alcohol free or sober.

We always stay *consistent* with our identity. If we identify as heavy drinkers, we'll do anything to get the next drink. And the opposite: If we change our identity to be a nondrinker, we'll do whatever it takes not to drink anymore.

You can see this during the night or on the morning after an evening when you've had more to drink than usual. You wake up feeling sick physically and frustrated with yourself, maybe asking again: *Why did I do this? Why do I keep drinking when I know it's bad for me?* And then you feel upset with yourself once again. You might think: *How am I loving myself fully when I keep making choices that aren't for the best and that let me and my body down? Something has to change.*

If we drink often and experience limiting hangovers, *we have only a little energy, willpower, and excitement to put toward our future. A great future requires planning, follow-through, creativity, energy, health, and more.* When we live as heavy drinkers, we accomplish a minimal part of what we want and lower our expectations of everything except our drink. We have only one life. Will you keep tolerating a dull future?

Self-Love and Self-Sabotage

Taking care of ourselves is fundamental to our well-being, allowing us to have a good life and preventing us from entering into negative situations, like self-sabotage. Self-sabotage is caused primarily when a person doubts her abilities; has substantial negative beliefs about the self; has fears linked to being judged; feels overwhelmed; or is in doubt about being able to meet expectations.

Another critical component that plays a role in self-sabotage is fear of success. In this case, what if we succeed in staying sober? How is leaving the comfort zone we have with alcohol going to feel? Will we lose fun, relaxation, relationships, social groups, and events? Many people start drinking again for this reason. The lack of self-control, or reduced self-control, can lead to challenges and stress with self-sabotaging behaviors.

> *"I'm 58 years old, and I've been dealing with self-sabotage related to alcohol for at least the last five years. My marriage ended painfully and has led to ongoing family issues—which I attribute entirely to myself, affecting my confidence and self-love. I tried to start a new relationship a few times, but all the men I met were losers, drunks, or narcissists. I thought, maybe I don't deserve better.*
>
> *"Around seven months ago, I decided to reduce my alcohol intake to two glasses a day. But because it's difficult for me to manage all these emotions when they reach a certain point, I forget that I'm trying to*

control my drinking. Then I engage in self-sabotaging by overdrinking for hours by myself or with friends, because I feel pressure to drink to fit in and be heard, especially when I want to talk about what I'm facing." —Alyssa

We can see that Alyssa's self-sabotaging using alcohol is a coping mechanism and a consequence of a combination of low self-confidence and self-love, fear of facing new situations, and peer pressure. She associates alcohol with momentary relief from these distressing feelings and forgets the high emotional and physical price she pays afterward when she realizes that she has to start all over again.

Identifying and addressing the causes that lead to self-sabotage are important. They connect with and influence how we act from impulses, without thinking, and have negative consequences for our identity, self-esteem, and the desired future we want to achieve.

Think about it...

Think about the last two or three self-sabotage episodes you've had and identify any patterns.

1. Are there any similarities in what happened or how you felt before, during, or after the episode?

2. By recognizing these patterns, can you develop a strategy to prevent a future self-sabotage event?

Self-sabotaging through using alcohol to avoid or cope with negative feelings creates *more problems in your life*. It's an exhausting road you might be taking. Going back and forth between overdrinking and staying sober can wear you out, *damaging you and your life right now and in the future.*

In conclusion, self-love is the foundation that empowers us to respect ourselves; to take care of our bodies, minds, and emotions; to make good decisions for our lives; to stop the toxic inputs (alcohol) and toxic relationships. With self-love, we will honor who we truly are as we become assertive with ourselves and in our relationships with others, create boundaries, go all in with what's good for us, and experience delight in who we are.

Notes:

CHAPTER 20

LOOKING FORWARD

No matter how careful you are about keeping your drinking in line,
or how far you have gone to the other side;
no matter how much control you have over your drinking,
or how bad your relationship with booze is right now,
you can find the way back to yourself.
It's in your hands to reconsider your drinking.
Now is the time.

Here we are, *you and us together at this point of the journey.* Thank you for trusting us until this last page. Becoming alcohol free is a major life change, and if you're here, it means that *you've decided to join us in living a more courageous and transformed life.*

Our purpose has been to give you the tools to reach this point of no return to your previous life—one in which you were unhappy and stuck in habits that were taking away the best of you. We've tried to show how misleading and destructive alcohol and the feminine drinking culture can be, making us believe we're part of something exciting, when, in reality, it's taking so much from us, reducing our possibilities and clouding our potential.

We know that you can return to your true and best self by following our method and workbook to make changes in your life—confronting your fears, learning what's necessary, and growing on a journey that can transform you. This includes looking at the world around you more critically and realizing that the pursuit of happiness is something much deeper than the false hopes and structure that alcohol seems to offer.

Grounding yourself in this new lifestyle will take continued courage, hard work, an open mind, and a positive mindset. Be encouraged by the strength you have as a woman! Time and again, research shows that women are psychologically stronger than men because of socialization skills and higher capacities to express emotions. These resources make us more resilient and better prepared to adjust to challenges.

Rescuing ourselves from our habit or addiction can be a transformative experience that enables and empowers us to move forward and improve our lives in extraordinary ways. Do it with a positive attitude. Honor yourself for prioritizing *you*, your health and future. With time, you'll come to enjoy and even love these changes and the new routines, experiences, and people you'll encounter on the journey.

As humans, we're constantly changing, even if we're not always conscious of it. But this time, *you have made the decision to change*, acting intentionally and with autonomy, and you have the *whys* and the *hows* for this change. What a privilege! Since it's an opportunity, be ready to act, to enjoy the experience; be grateful for the chance to transform yourself. *The time is now.*

As many times as you need to, and especially when you face challenges, return to your center, with respect and appreciation, and take the next small step available to continue your journey of expanding your life. We invite you to come back to the resources and ideas in this book any time and to apply them to other areas in your life as well.

With the clarity you have gained from reading our book and working on these steps of change with us, with trust in yourself, with renewed clarity and positive feelings, build a new present and future for yourself and your loved ones.

With all the advantages of being in the driver's seat of your life, your future is bright!

Notes:

APPENDIX

Disclaimer: These quizzes are the product of clinical observations intended for conjecture purposes only. The questions and results provided in these quizzes have yet to undergo validation through formal research or scientific study. Therefore, the accuracy and reliability of the outcomes may vary. Participants are encouraged to interpret the results with discretion and not rely on them as definitive assessments. The creators of these quizzes advise users to consult qualified professionals for any serious inquiries or concerns. By participating in these quizzes, users acknowledge and accept these terms.

QUIZ #1

What is your relationship with alcohol?

Instructions:

Respond to each question with 1, 2 or 3 points.

1 Point: Rarely
2 Points: Sometimes
3 Points: Always

1. I think of having a drink as soon as I get home, no matter what time it is.	
2. I have a lot of anticipation and excitement about drinking.	
3. I can drink for long periods of time, and I think I developed a high tolerance.	
4. I feel I drink too much, and I may have experienced problems with my children, spouse, friends and extended family.	
5. I can't imagine myself being sober/alcohol-free, as I don't like sober people.	
6. I like to drink when I am happy and also when I am depressed, anxious, or under stress.	

7. I have set routines around my drinking; for example, a specific time of the day, a particular place, using a favorite glass. I don't plan any other activities around those times; my drinking is a priority.	
8. I have good times while drinking and can't imagine a day or social event without it.	
9. I want to drink when I am by myself. It's my "me" time	
10. I plan to have enough alcohol. I may forget other important things, but I will never be out of alcohol at home.	
11. I feel happy when I start drinking, and I hope I will be in control.	
12. After I crossed the line (during the night or the next day), I promise myself to control my drinking in the future.	
13. I had a flash of clarity about drinking too much. I don't like what I saw about me and my future, but then I forget about that and keep drinking the same.	
14. I feel that I drink too much; I wonder if I will have health conditions due to my drinking.	

15. I feel I can trust that I'll drink in moderation in the future, but I don't always follow through.	
16. I have experienced binge drinking (defined as four or more drinks in two hours) in the past month.	
17. I love my drinking buddies, and I want to hang out with them as much as possible, at times maybe more than my kids, spouse, and family.	
18. I am more outgoing and assertive when I have a drink. I like my "tipsy" personality.	
19. I don't tell the truth about how much I drink to my spouse, closest family, and friends.	
20. I experience hangovers at least once a week.	
21. Even if I have been drinking too much, I feel that I can drive myself back home.	
Total	

Interpretation

Low Score (0-15): Casual Relationship

You may have a *casual relationship* with alcohol if you drink, but alcohol isn't important in your life. Crossing the line would be rare but possible in the long term. Just as a relationship with an acquaintance can grow over time as you see the person more frequently, the same can happen with alcohol; the relationship can move from casual to central. So, think about the consequences when you start drinking often.

Medium Score (16-36): Central Relationship

You may have a *central relationship* with alcohol in which drinking is vital: Alcohol is part of your daily routine. Every occasion is suitable for a drink, and all your social activities revolve around alcohol consumption. Nevertheless, you may not consider that you *already have* an alcohol problem except for an occasional flash of clarity. As your relationship with alcohol becomes closer, issues arise in your other relationships. Still, they are transient and may be mended in the short term in most cases.

High Score (37-63): Committed Relationship

You might be in a *committed relationship* with alcohol. You feel firmly attached to your drink, with signs of substantial psychological and emotional dependence. Being in this relationship will make you overdrink every day and cross the line consistently. You and your drink live together, and all other relationships and realities take second place. This type of dependency creates a profound change in your life. You may start having difficulties with your job, family, and health as you become self-absorbed with your drink. Alcohol will turn out to be your primary commitment or priority.

QUIZ #2

Are you part of the feminine drinking culture?

The feminine drinking culture (FDC) tells women: *"Having a drink is your right. You earned it. You deserve it. You need it. Drinking alcohol is part of our bond."*

1. Ask yourself: *How do I see alcohol?* Think about it, and check your responses to the following questions:

How do you see alcohol?
- ☐ It's a fun habit ("wine o'clock"), not an addiction.
- ☐ It makes me more outgoing, extroverted, easygoing and fun.
- ☐ In certain situations (e.g., girls' nights), heavy drinking is not only accepted but also expected.
- ☐ It's legal, not a drug.
- ☐ It's a way to connect with my social circles and deepen my friendships.
- ☐ It's an essential component of all social activities; drinking is the norm.
- ☐ It's a way to release multiple pressures and decompress.
- ☐ It's a way to reward myself; I deserve to enjoy life, to be happy.
- ☐ I believe that alcohol is synonymous with fun.
- ☐ I think I have my drinking under control but sometimes I don't follow through because of special situations.
- ☐ I drink to relax, let everything go, untangle something, calm down, ease the strain.
- ☐ I work hard all day doing things for others, why shouldn't I have something for myself?

☐ I drink to keep up with colleagues and friends.
☐ I have to drink on date nights.
☐ Sober sex lacks passion.

Count the number of responses you checked:

- 1–3 You are not part of the feminine drinking culture.
- 4–15 You are part of the feminine drinking culture.

BIBLIOGRAPHY

American College of Lifestyle Medicine (ACLM). "6 Ways to Take Control of Your Health: Lifestyle Medicine," *ACLM,* 2023, accessed May 5, 2023, https://lifestylemedicine.org/wp-content/uploads/2023/06/Pillar-Booklet.pdf.

American Psychiatric Association (2013).

Centers for Disease Control and Prevention (CDC). "Alcohol and Public Health: Frequently Asked Questions," *CDC,* last reviewed April 19, 2022, accessed May 2023, https://www.cdc.gov/alcohol/faqs.htm.

CDC. "Deaths from Excessive Alcohol Use in the United States," *CDC,* last reviewed July 6, 2022, accessed May 5, 2023, https://www.cdc.gov/alcohol/features/excessive-alcohol-deaths.html.

CDC. "Effects of Drinking Alcohol on Your Health," *CDC: Alcohol Portal,* page last reviewed September 14, 2022, accessed May 5, 2023, https://www.cdc.gov/alcoholportal/.

CDC. "Excessive Alcohol Use Is a Risk to Women's Health," *CDC,* last reviewed October 17, 2022, accessed May 2023, https://www.cdc.gov/alcohol/fact-sheets/womens-health.htm.

Daviet, Remi, Gokhan Aydogan, Kanchana Jagannathan, Nathaniel Spilka, Philipp D. Koellinger, Henry R. Kranzler et al. "Associations between

Alcohol Consumption and Gray and White Matter Volumes in the UK Biobank," *Nature Communications* 13, no 1 (March 4, 2022): 1–11, https://doi.org/10.1038/s41467-022-28735-5.

Gilligan, Conor, and Kypros Kypri. "Parent Attitudes, Family Dynamics and Adolescent Drinking: Qualitative Study of the Australian Parenting Guidelines for Adolescent Alcohol Use," *BMC Public Health* 12 (2012): 7.

Granfield, Robert, and William Cloud. *Coming Clean: Overcoming Addiction without Treatment* (New York: New York University Press, 1999).

Hayes, Louise, Diana Smart, John W. Toumbourou, and Ann Sanson. "Parenting Influences on Adolescent Use," *Australian Institute of Family Studies* (2004): 70.

Johnston, Ann D. *Drink: The Intimate Relationship between Women and Alcohol* (Harper Wave, 2013).

Knapp, Caroline. *Drinking: A Love Story* (New York: The Dial Press, 1996).

Koob, George F., "Keynote: 'Alcohol and the Female Brain,'" *2017 National Conference on Alcohol and Opioid Use in Women and Girls: Advances in Prevention, Treatment and Recovery Research*, presented October 27, 2017.

Koob, George F. and Nora D. Volkow, "Neurobiology of Addiction: A Neurocircuitry Analysis," *The Lancet Psychiatry* 3, no. 8 (August 2016): 760–773.

Kubler-Ross, Elisabeth, and David Kessler. *On Grief and Grieving* (Simon and Schuster, 2014).

Loscalzo, Joseph, Anthony Fauci, Dennis Kasper, Stephen Hauser, Dan Longo, and J. Larry Jameson, *Harrison's Principles of Internal Medicine*, 21st ed., (McGraw Hill, 2022).

Merriam-Webster.com Dictionary. S.v. "hair of the dog (that bit you)," accessed August 7, 2023, https://www.merriam-webster.com/dictionary/hair%20of%20the%20dog%20%28that%20bit%20you%29.

National Drug and Alcohol Research Centre (NDARC). "Parents May Be Putting Their Children on a Path to Drinking," *NDARC,* published September 8, 2014, accessed August 2023, https://ndarc.med.unsw.edu.au/news/parents-may-be-putting-their-children-path-drinking.

National Institute on Alcohol Abuse and Alcoholism (NIAAA). "What Are the U.S. Guidelines for Drinking?" *NIAAA,* accessed July 2023, https://www.rethinkingdrinking.niaaa.nih.gov/how-much-is-too-much/is-your-drinking-pattern-risky/Drinking-Levels.aspx#:~:text=descargar%20el%20documento-,What%20are%20the%20U.S.%20guidelines%20for%20drinking%3F,women%20when%20alcohol%20is%20consumed.

NIAAA. "Alcohol Effects on Health: Research-Based Information on Drinking and Its Impact," *NIAAA,* accessed May 5, 2023, https://www.niaaa.nih.gov/alcohols-effects-health.

NIAAA. "Women and Alcohol," *NIAAA,* updated March 2023, accessed May 2023, https://www.niaaa.nih.gov/publications/brochures-and-fact-sheets/women-and-alcohol.

Pollard, Michael, Joan S. Tucker, and Harold D. Green Jr. "Changes in Adult Alcohol Use and Consequences during the COVID-19 Pandemic in the US," *JAMA Network Open* 3, no. 9 (September 29, 2020), doi:10.1001/jamanetworkopen.2020.22942.

Retzinger, Suzanne M. "Resentment and Laughter: Video Studies of the Shame-Rage Spiral," in *The Role of Shame in Symptom Formation*, ed. Helen B. Lewis, (Hillsdale, NJ: Erlbaum, 1987): 151–181.

Slade, Tim, Cath Chapman, and Maree Teeson. "Women's Alcohol Consumption Catching up to Men: Why This Matters," *NDARC*, accessed July 2023, https://ndarc.med.unsw.edu.au/blog/womens-alcohol-consumption-catching-men-why-matters.

Slade, Tim, Cath Chapman, Wendy Swift, Katherine Keyes, Zoe Tonks, and Maree Teeson. "Birth Cohort Trends in the Global Epidemiology of Alcohol Use and Alcohol-Related Harms in Men and Women: Systematic Review and Metaregression," *BMJ Open* 6, no. 10 (October 24, 2016):e011827, doi: 10.1136/bmjopen-2016-011827.

Steele, Claude M., and Robert A. Josephs, "Alcohol Myopia: Its Prized and Dangerous Effects." *American Psychologist*, 45 (1990): 921–933.

Stuewig, Jeffrey, June P. Tangney, Caron Heigel, Laura Harty, and Laura McCloskey. "Shaming, Blaming, and Maiming: Functional Links among the Moral Emotions, Externalization of Blame, and Aggression," *Journal of Research in Personality* 44, no. 1 (February 1, 2010): 91–102. doi: 10.1016/j.jrp.2009.12.005. PMID: 20369025; PMCID: PMC2848360.

White, Aaron M. "Gender Differences in the Epidemiology of Alcohol Use and Related Harms in United States," *Alcohol Research Current Reviews* 40, no. 2, accessed May 2023, https://arcr.niaaa.nih.gov/volume/40/2/gender-differences-epidemiology-alcohol-use-and-related-harms-united-states.

White, Aaron M., I-Jen P. Castle, Ralph W. Hingson, and Patricia A. Powell, "Using Death Certificates to Explore Changes in Alcohol-Related Mortality in the United States, 1999 to 2017," Alcoholism: Clinical and Experimental Research 44, no. 1 (January 7, 2020): 178-187, https://doi.org/10.1111/acer.14239.

White, Aaron, I-Jen P Castle, Chiung M. Chen, Mariela Shirley, Deidra Roach, and Ralph Hingson. "Converging Patterns of Alcohol Use and

Related Outcomes among Females and Males in the United States, 2002 to 2012," *Alcoholism: Clinical and Experimental Research* 39, no. 9 (September 2015):1712–26. PMID: 26331879.

World Heart Federation (WHF). "The Impact of Alcohol on Cardiovascular Health: Myths and Measures," *WHF*, published January 20, 2022, accessed May 2023, https://world-heart-federation.org/news/no-amount-of-alcohol-is-good-for-the-heart-says-world-heart-federation/.

Yeomans, Martin R., Samantha Caton, and Marion M. Hetherington. "Alcohol and Food Intake," *Current Opinion in Clinical Nutrition and Metabolic Care* 6, no. 6 (November 2023): 639–644, doi: 10.1097/00075197-200311000-00006. PMID: 14557794.

ACKNOWLEDGEMENTS

During our journey of a comprehensive exploration of the complicated relationship between women and alcohol, we constantly received an overwhelming wave of interest and support from those with whom we shared our project. Witnessing the enthusiasm and curiosity that greeted our undertaking was genuinely heartening. We extend our gratitude to the individuals with whom we spoke from diverse corners of the globe—from the vibrant cultures of Central and South America to the rich tapestry of Asia, the storied history of Europe, and the melting pot of perspectives found in the United States.

Among our supporters were colleagues whose insights enriched our discussions, friends who lent their relentless encouragement, and acquaintances of acquaintances whose interests sparked enlightening exchanges. These conversations unfolded in various settings—from chance encounters in airports, parks, trips, parties, dinners, and also during moments of reflection in the dynamic atmosphere of conferences. Even amidst the hustle and bustle of networking events, the passion for our topic sparked.

We owe our gratitude to everyone who expressed interest in our work. Your collective curiosity provided us with the inspiration, energy, and discipline to continue and reaffirmed to us the importance of this topic. It is with genuine appreciation that we acknowledge the role you played in shaping and sustaining our journey.

We extend our deepest gratitude to our beloved and cheerful **family**, whose support and encouragement have been invaluable throughout our writing journey. They have generously shared their time and attention, offered candid feedback, and stood by us during the most challenging moments of this endeavor. Each member has been a genuine and caring companion in our shared adventure of navigating uncharted territories where there was no path; the path was made by walking. Special thanks to Dr. William Triplett for his significant contributions to the medical contents of the book.

We are deeply grateful to our friend, **Susana Rigato**, who was one of the first readers of the manuscript. Her firm personal support, assistance, and network connections were invaluable throughout this endeavor. Susana's directness and approachability made our conversations enjoyable and productive as we navigated the process of writing this book. Susana's encouragement and companionship on this singular journey were immensely appreciated and will always be remembered with gratitude.

In the journey of crafting this work, we were fortunate to have the presence of our friend **Walt Locke**, who was also one of the first readers of the manuscript. From the earliest stages of conception to the final moments of refinement, Walt stood by us, offering a shoulder to lean on and a source of laughter and joy. Beyond the warmth of his friendship, Walt shared his wisdom and insight, offering guidance and advice. Thank you for believing in us and infusing our journey with love, laughter, and light.

Acknowledgements

Rosemary Daniell stood alongside us from the very start, both as an expert reader and within the dynamic circle of the **Zona Rosa sisters**. We owe a debt of gratitude to her for her enduring presence and invaluable contributions. In recognizing her pivotal role, we also extend our heartfelt appreciation to her sisterhood, each adding their unique touch to our shared path. Rosemary's commitment and camaraderie have truly enriched our experience. We extend our most profound appreciation for the consistent encouragement, constructive critiques, and unwavering support we have received from all those involved, especially from Rosemary.

Nicole Gardiner played a crucial role in the development of this project, offering invaluable ideas and innovative suggestions from the earliest stages of conception through to the final moments of refinement. Nicole's support and belief in the project's potential kept us motivated and inspired throughout the journey. She provided us with insights, helping us navigate complex challenges with her wisdom and practical advice. We are deeply grateful for her dedication, as her efforts significantly enriched the quality and success of our work.

We present our gratitude to our editor **Olivia Bauer**, whose firm dedication and exceptional editorial skills have been instrumental in finishing this book. She provided guidance and, insightful feedback. Olivia's keen eye for detail, coupled with a *profound understanding of our vision*, has significantly enhanced the manuscript's clarity, coherence, and overall quality. Her willingness to go above and beyond has made this journey productive and immensely rewarding.

We want to extend our sincere gratitude to **Bethany Kelly** and her team at **Publishing Partner** for their invaluable contributions to this project. From the initial stages to the final delivery of the book into your hands, they have consistently demonstrated professionalism, expertise, and a remarkable ability to simplify even the most challenging tasks. Her ability to easily navigate complex chores ensured a smooth journey from conception to completion. We are truly grateful for her invaluable support and expertise, which made the seemingly impossible possible.

Our heartfelt gratitude to each and every person who has been a source of inspiration, encouragement, and support in bringing this book to completion. Your sound support has been instrumental in shaping not only the pages of this book but also our current mission. We are deeply thankful for all you've provided throughout this journey.

ABOUT THE AUTHORS

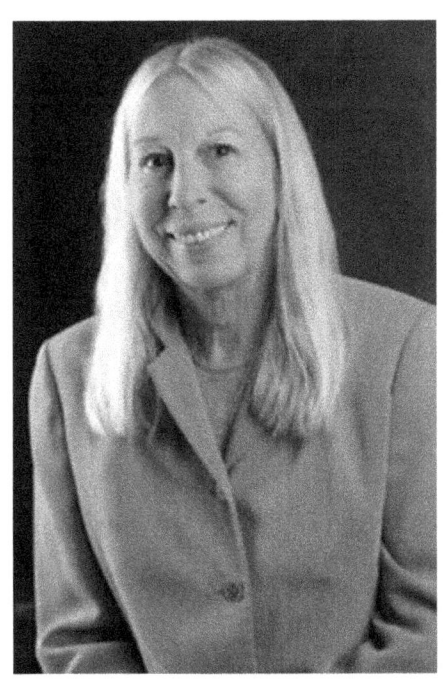

Alicia Lamberghini-West, PsyD, is a Licensed Clinical Psychologist and Published Author. She has twenty-five years of experience in Psychiatric Rehabilitation and private practice with a strong focus on women's issues. Established as a global expert, advisor, therapist, presenter, and lecturer on various topics surrounding mental health, addictions, and gender subjects, she integrates American and International clinical practice and research into effective strategies for women navigating social pressures, limitations, and complicated gender issues. Dr. Lamberghini-West possesses a lifelong passion for empowering women in all aspects of their lives—across cultures, ages, and social classes, being a well-known expert in rehabilitation involving the challenges women face. She is on the Fulbright Specialist Roster for this subject. In 2019 she published *Your Life, Your Way: Become Aware of Social Pressures Limiting Women*.

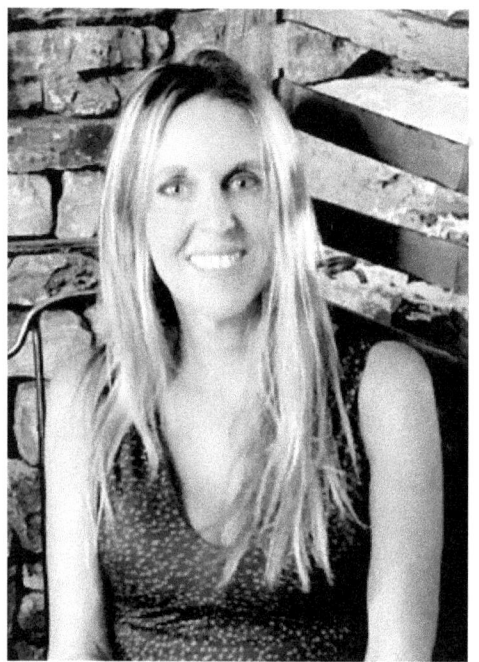

Pilar Karlen Triplett was born in Buenos Aires, Argentina. She has lived in the USA for 20 years and has a successful Life and Health Coach practice, focusing on Total Life Transformation. She has also been an engineer for 27 years, and she applies her engineering mindset and logic systems to her holistic coaching practice. Her innovative method offers her clients a new way to transform their lives.

Dr. William Triplett is a board-certified family medicine physician with over 23 years of experience in primary care, acute care and military medicine. He is a retired USAF and Air National Guard flight surgeon. He possesses a keen and growing interest in substance abuse and addiction and has advocated a sober lifestyle to his patients for many years. He lives in the Missouri Ozarks with his wife Pilar and dog Luna Bear, where he enjoys hiking, swimming, kayaking, and cooking.

www.ingramcontent.com/pod-product-compliance
Lightning Source LLC
Chambersburg PA
CBHW052028030426
42337CB00027B/4905